Telehealth

Edited by Thomas F. Heston

Published in London, United Kingdom

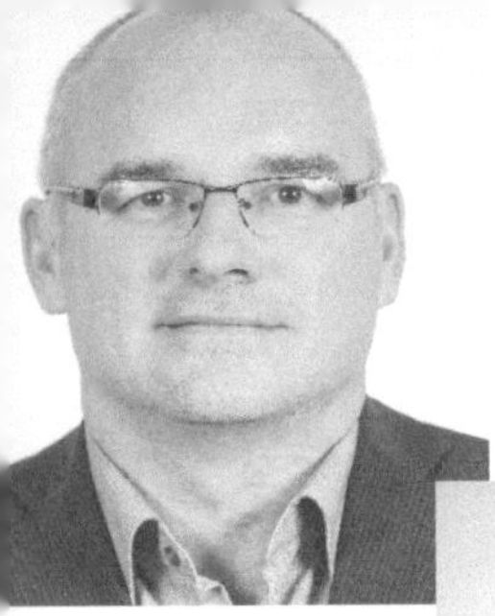
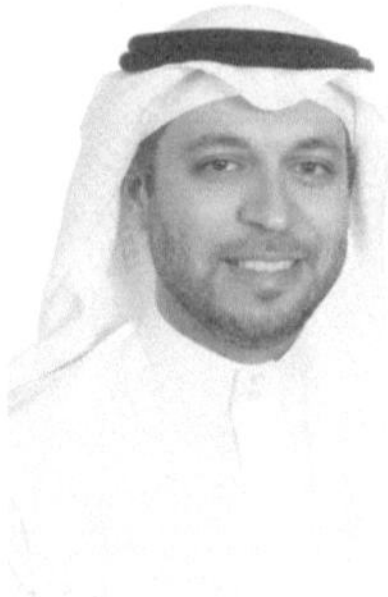
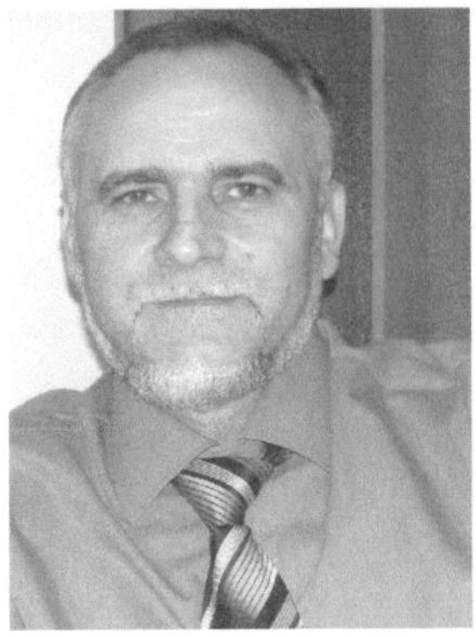
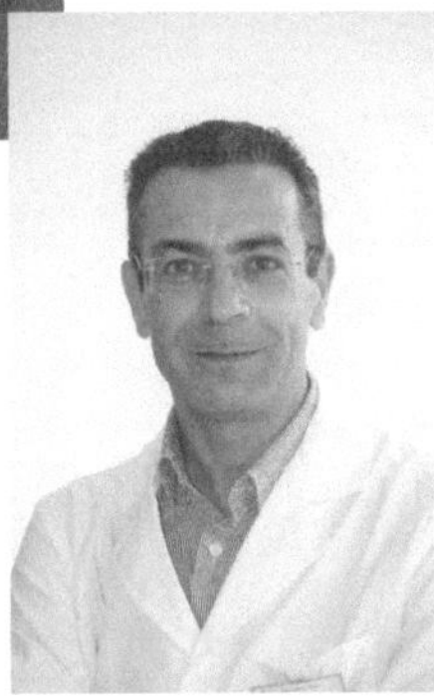
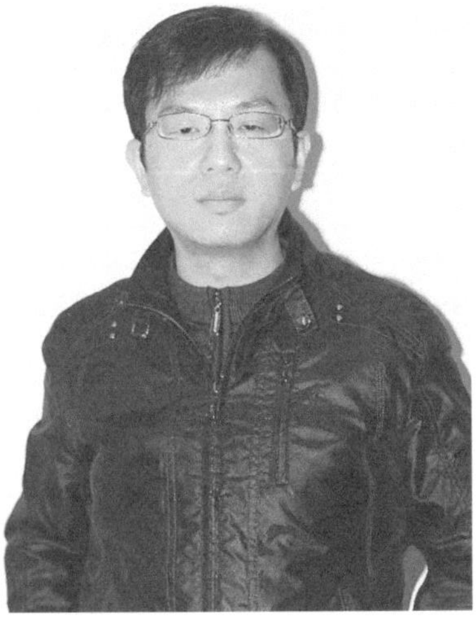
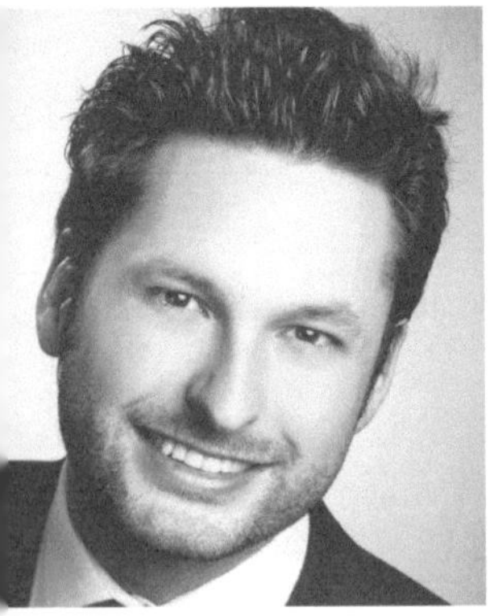
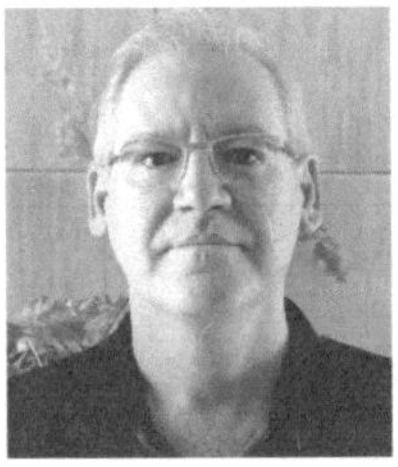

IntechOpen

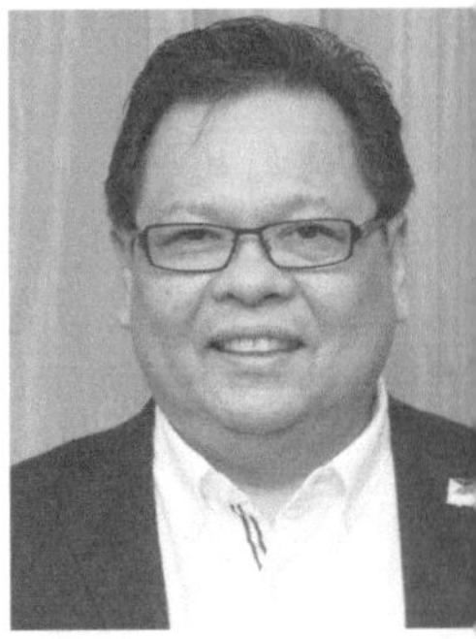
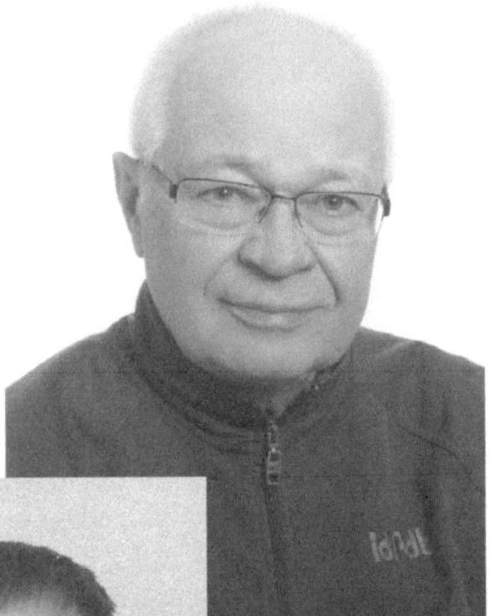
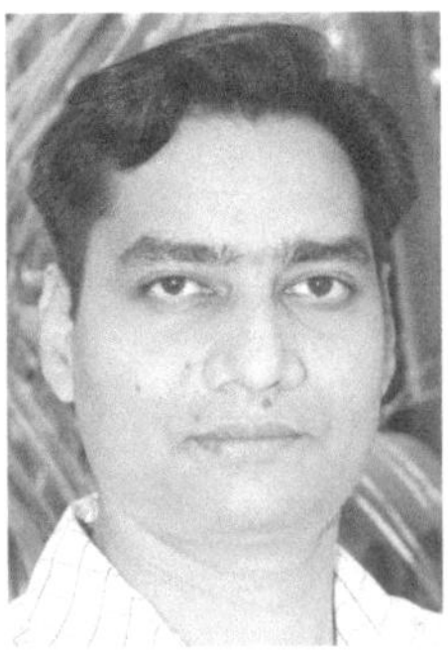
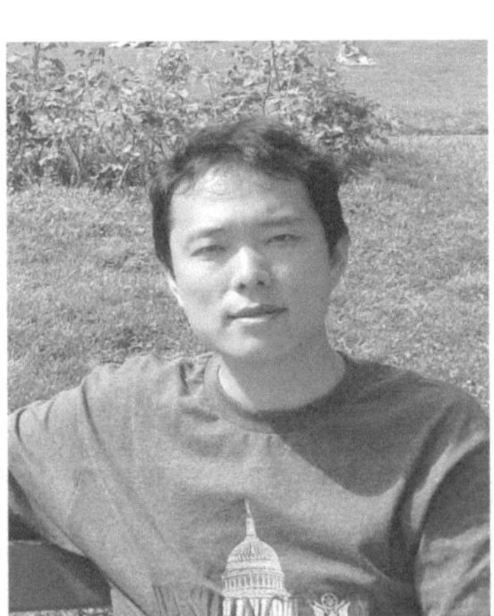
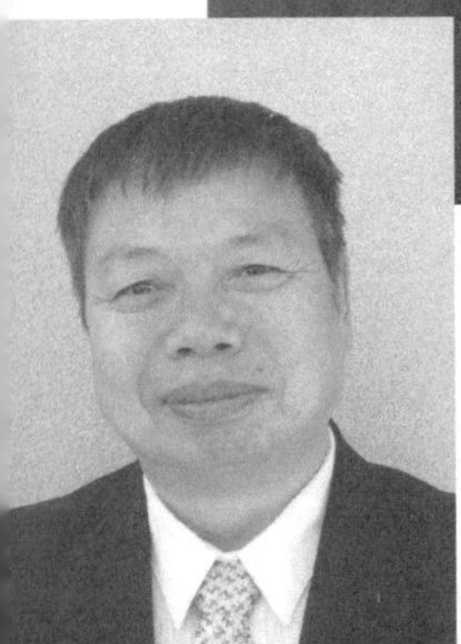
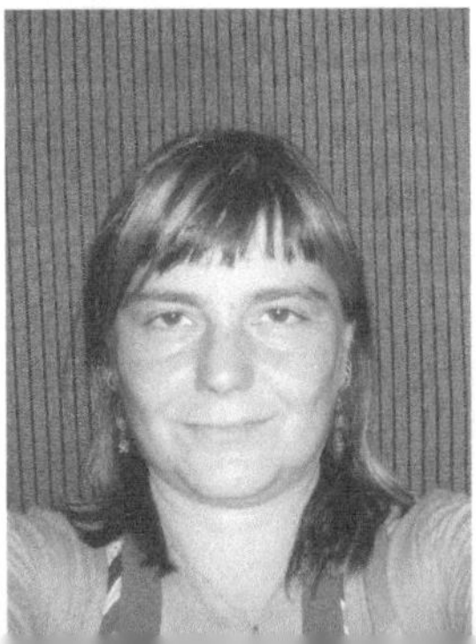

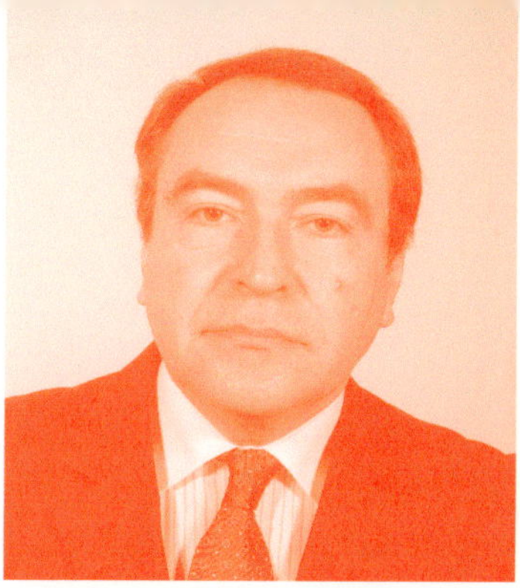
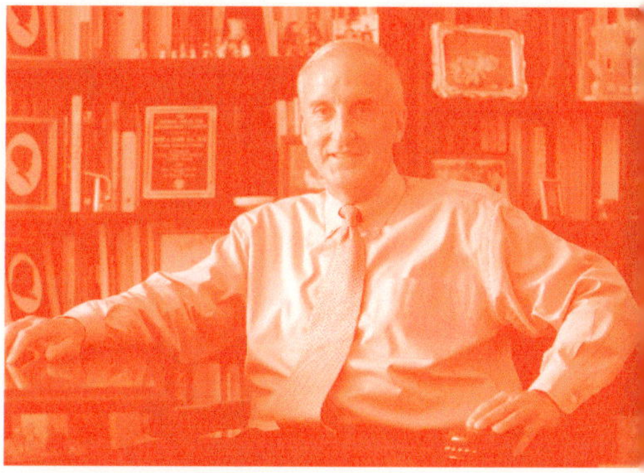
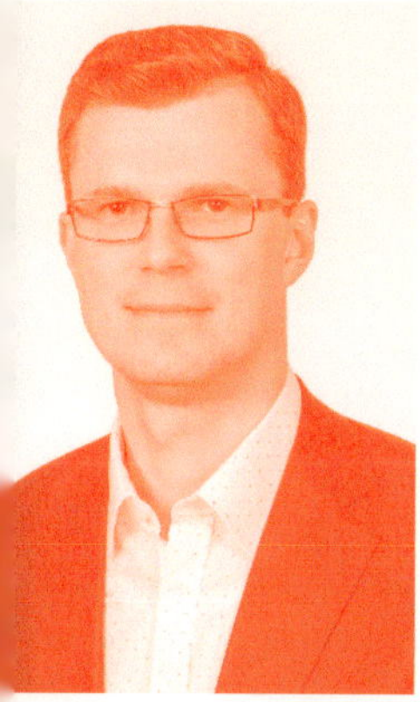
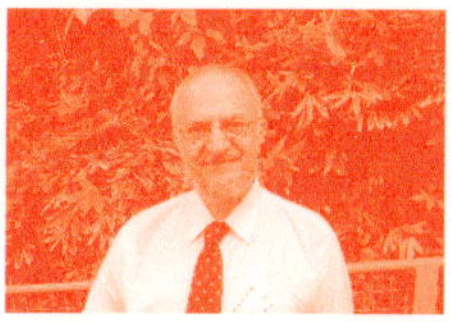
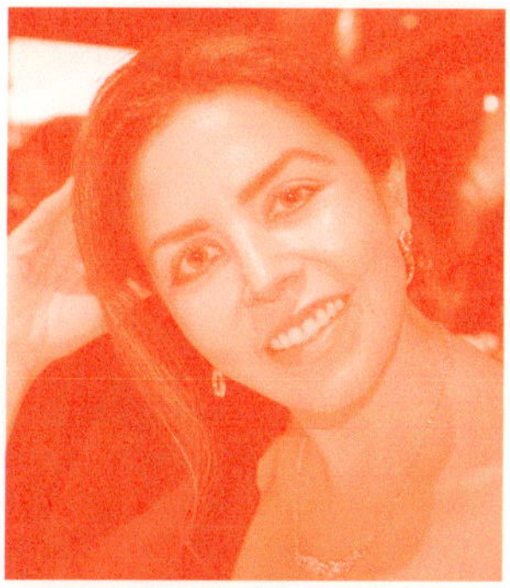

Supporting open minds since 2005

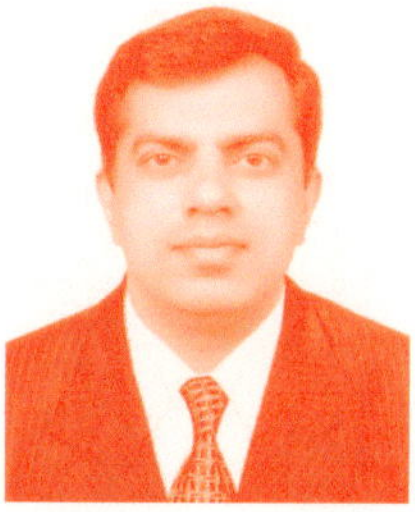
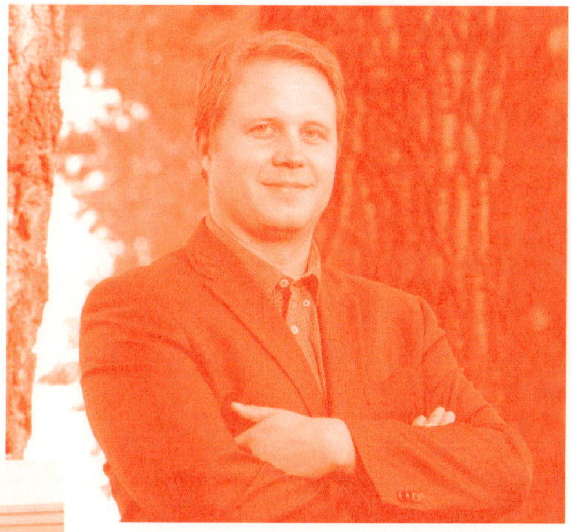
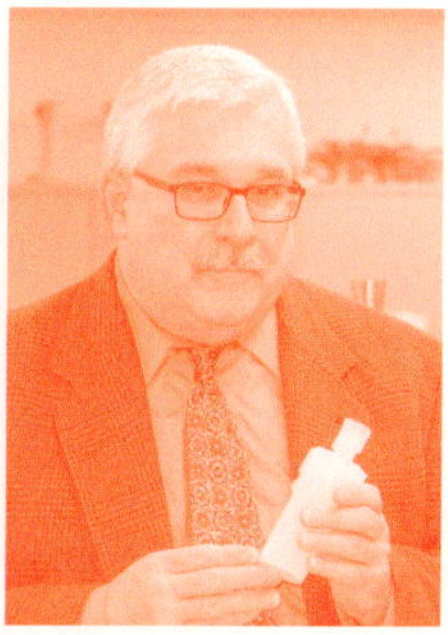
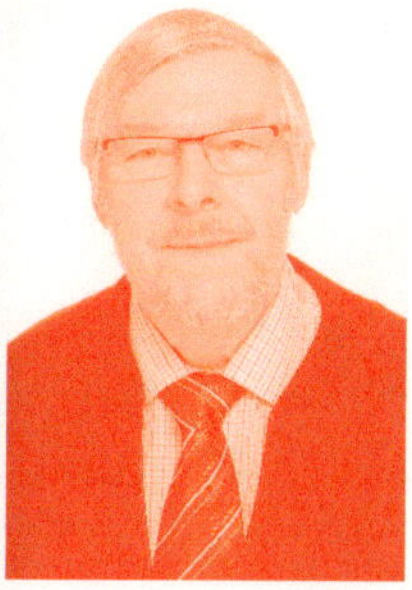
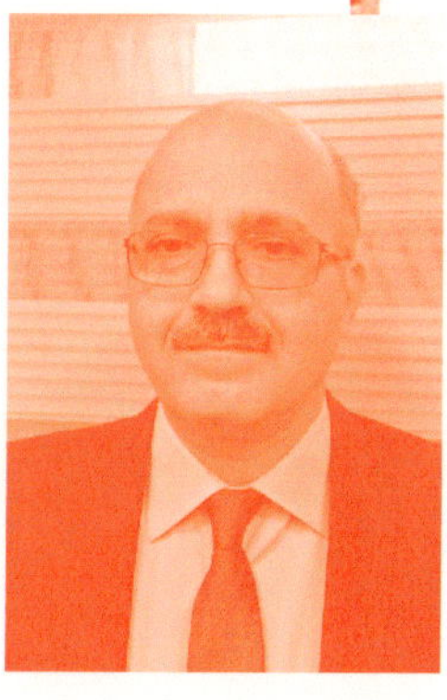
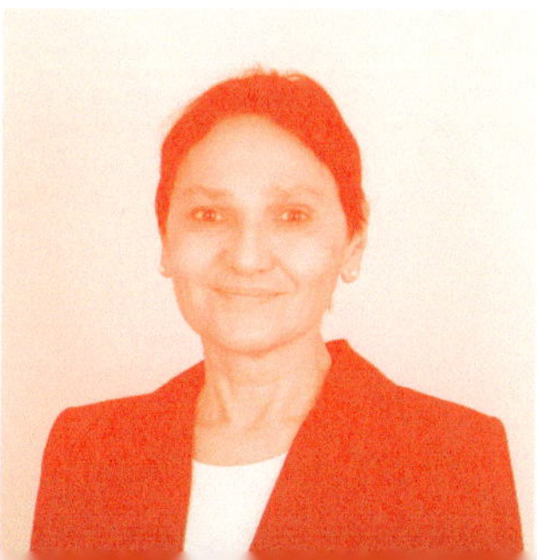
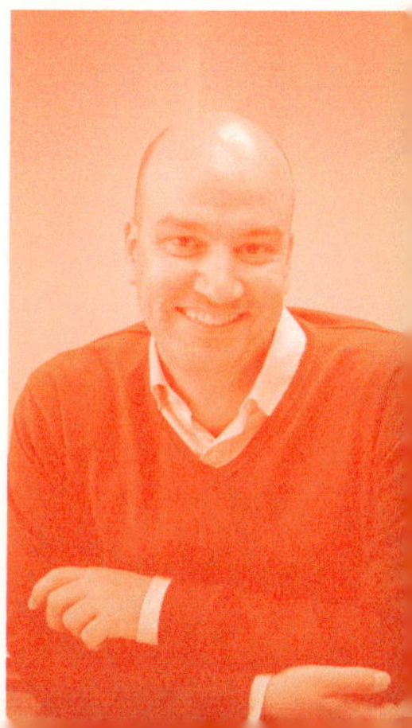

Telehealth
http://dx.doi.org/10.5772/intechopen.78461
Edited by Thomas F. Heston

Contributors
Jian-Chiun Liou, Surya Bali, Ahmad Hoirul Basori, Hani Moaiteq Abdullah AlJahdali, Antonio Rienzo, Thomas F. Heston

First published in London, United Kingdom, 2019 by IntechOpen
IntechOpen is the global imprint of INTECHOPEN LIMITED, registered in England and Wales, registration number: 11086078, The Shard, 25th floor, 32 London Bridge Street
London, SE19SG – United Kingdom
Printed in Croatia

British Library Cataloguing-in-Publication Data
A catalogue record for this book is available from the British Library

Additional hard copies can be obtained from orders@intechopen.com

Telehealth
Edited by Thomas F. Heston
p. cm.
Print ISBN 978-1-78985-497-8
Online ISBN 978-1-78985-498-5

Meet the editor

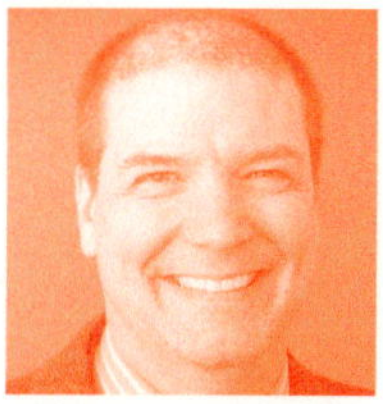

Dr. Thomas F. Heston is a practicing physician and clinical Associate Professor at the Elson S. Floyd College of Medicine in Spokane, Washington, USA. As a nuclear medicine resident in the early 1990s he researched the application of neural networks in transplant medicine. He subsequently started the first nuclear medicine teleradiology network to rural northern Idaho, and in the process developed the picture archiving and communication system for the network. He then went on to study positron emission tomography (PET) at Johns Hopkins University. As an assistant professor (adjunct) at Johns Hopkins, he established the first PET/computed tomography program in the United Arab Emirates cancer center in Al Ain. His current research focus is on the application of blockchain technology to health care.

Contents

Preface

This first edition of *Telehealth* provides readers with an introduction to the latest developments in the remote practice of medicine. Telemedicine allows specialized medical care to even the most remote and underserved regions of the world not only by facilitating voice communication but also by enabling remote physical diagnosis using advanced robotic technology. This book on telemedicine provides the reader with an overview of some of the latest developments in the field of telemedicine. There remains much work to do to realize the great potential of telemedicine. These chapters will give readers a good start.

Thomas F. Heston, MD, FAAFP, FASNC, FACNM
Clinical Associate Professor,
Elson S. Floyd College of Medicine,
Washington State University,
Spokane, Washington USA

Section 1

Introduction

Chapter 1

Introductory Chapter: Telemedicine

Thomas F. Heston

1. Introduction

The practice of telemedicine creates opportunities for greater access to medical care, improved access to medical specialists, and greater convenience for patients, all at a potentially lower financial cost. With the global expansion of the Internet via cable, fiber optics, satellites, drones, and even high altitude balloons, telemedicine services can reach every individual on Earth with a smartphone.

2. History of telemedicine

Telemedicine in its earliest form began with the advent of the telegraph in 1844 and the telephone in 1876, which allowed patients to summon physicians quickly and increased the availability of physician-to-physician consultations [1]. During the American Civil War, the telegraph was used to transmit casualty lists and request medical supplies. After the telegraphy, telephones were developed and became the primary means of remote medical communication. The use of portable radios became common starting in the early 1900s. The National Aeronautics and Space Administration (NASA) revolutionized long-distance communications in the mid to late 1900s by developing systems to both communicate with and monitor the health of astronauts. With increasing technology including computing and telecommunication over the Internet, telemedicine has grown to include real-time remote consultation from medical specialists, remote access to medical imaging, home monitoring of patients, and increased availability of patient as well as physician medical education resources [2].

3. Current status

Applications of telemedicine continue to grow rapidly. Current applications have advanced to the point that in addition to physicians monitoring patients remotely there are artificial intelligence systems using smartphones and wearable applications to monitor patient health [3]. Not only does telemedicine allow advanced verbal communication between physicians and patients, it also enables physicians to conduct a physical exam of patients remotely and to even conduct surgery over long distances using telerobotic systems [4].

4. Future developments and challenges

Telemedicine attempts to replicate the patient-to-doctor relationship in a realistic, productive manner. Transmitting sensory data over the Internet presents a primary challenge to the practice of telemedicine [5]. Lack of awareness and experience with the technology, along with uncertainties over how telemedical

IntechOpen

services will be reimbursed, have limited the expansion of telemedicine in spite of its great promise [6]. In addition, the quality of medical services offered over some commercial telemedicine services can vary widely. For example, one study looking at the medical diagnosis and management of skin disorders via telemedicine found that several diagnoses were consistently missed (secondary syphilis, eczema herpeticum, Gram-negative folliculitis, and polycystic ovarian syndrome) and common diagnoses that were correctly made were often incorrectly treated [7]. Familiarity with technology and comfort with the use of smartphones and healthcare apps also appears to be a primary challenge facing the implementation of telemedicine. For example, Millennials, who have grown up with the Internet and smartphones, are much more interested in using healthcare apps and telemedicine services compared to baby boomers [8]. As technology becomes more user-friendly, people become more comfortable with technology, and as smartphones become widely available, telemedicine will continue to show rapid development. The authors in this book on telemedicine are leading the way!

Author details

Thomas F. Heston[1,2]

1 Department of Medical Education and Clinical Sciences, Elson S. Floyd College of Medicine, Washington State University, Spokane, Washington, USA

2 Department of Behavioral Sciences, International American University, St. Lucia

*Address all correspondence to: tomhestonmd@gmail.com

References

[1] Cipolat C, Geiges M. The history of telemedicine. In: Burg G, editor. Telemedicine and Teledermatology. Basel: Karger; 2002. pp. 6-11

[2] Zundel KM. Telemedicine: History, applications, and impact on librarianship. Bulletin of the Medical Library Association. 1996;**84**(1):71-79

[3] Kelly D, Curran K, Caulfield B. Automatic prediction of health status using smartphone-derived behavior profiles. IEEE Journal of Biomedical and Health Informatics. 2017;**21**(6):1750-1760

[4] Avgousti S, Christoforou EG, Panayides AS, Voskarides S, Novales C, Nouaille L, et al. Medical telerobotic systems: Current status and future trends. Biomedical Engineering Online. 2016;**15**(1):96

[5] Lupton D, Maslen S. Telemedicine and the senses: A review. Sociology of Health & Illness. 2017;**39**(8):1557-1571

[6] Farr C. Why Telemedicine has been a Bust [Internet]. CNBC. 2018. Available from: https://www.cnbc.com/2018/06/29/why-telemedicine-is-a-bust.html [Cited: November 1, 2018]

[7] Resneck JS, Abrouk M, Steuer M, Tam A, Yen A, Lee I, et al. Choice, transparency, coordination, and quality among direct-to-consumer telemedicine websites and apps treating skin disease. JAMA Dermatology. 2016;**152**(7):768-775

[8] Sanborn BJ. Millennials Demand Telehealth in a Move Away From Traditional Primary Care Model [Internet]. Health IT News. 2018. Available from: https://www.healthcareitnews.com/news/millennials-demand-telehealth-move-away-traditional-primary-care-model [Cited: November 3, 2018]

Section 2

New Developments

Chapter 2

An Analysis of Telemedicine Experiences and Services in Chile

Antonio Rienzo Renato

Abstract

Applications based on telemedicine have been progressively increasing, and Chile is not the exception. After a set of isolated projects and government programs, a National Telehealth Program has been defined in the country. The content of this chapter intends to make a contribution to know the current situation of the country in this area. The author explains the main reasons why there is inequity, and geographic and demographic conditions that drive the need for this type of telemedical applications to grant and improve the health care of the population are explained. The chapter includes a brief theoretical conceptual summary with the characteristics, advantages, and disadvantages that telemedicine incorporates. Also, he presents the results of some of his investigations. Finally, the foundations and lines of action of the new Telehealth program that has been launched in the country are presented.

Keywords: telemedicine, Telehealth, e-health, telemedicine services, home care, information and communication technologies (ICTs)

1. Introduction

One of the major problems defined by the World Health Organization (WHO) in patient satisfaction is precisely not being satisfied with the system. Long waiting times to find a solution to their pathologies and long waiting lists to be able to perform exams or surgery are the problems that bare the lack of implementation and lack of specialists within the public service. In addition, if we add the evolution of the population toward an aging population as projected by the United Nations, where according to data from the 2017 revision of the report "Perspectives of World Population," it is expected that the number of people over 60 or more years (13% of the world population) will double by 2050 and triple by 2100; it will go from 962 million in 2017 to 2100 million in 2050 and 3100 million in 2100, reaching 22% [1, 2]. This population is more prone to chronic and degenerative diseases, which entail a wide demand for beds and days of hospitalization in the public service, which obviously makes the situation of overpopulation of patients in hospitals worse; attacking these diseases in a preventative manner, with monitoring systems, and country level strategies of care and prevention would be ideal to reduce the cases of chronic patients, assuming the aging of the population, but at the same time taking it with full responsibility in the field of public health.

On the other hand, in the context of Chile, we have a country with a unique topography, between the Andes mountain range on one side and the Pacific Ocean on the other, with a width of only 177 km from east to west and 5152 km from north to south, where the population is poorly distributed with an average country density of 20.4 Hab/km^2, but with some cities having more than 400 Hab/km^2, we have a collapsed system [3]. Therefore, doctors and specialists are concentrated in cities with higher densities, thus, causing a great social and economic cost for patients from more isolated sectors who must go to the major centers of reference to receive medical care. This is why the country is in an unbeatable position to allocate resources and be a leader in applications that help to decongest hospitals, decrease waiting lists, and grant access to the inhabitants of more isolated areas in our country. Telemedicine is considered as a solution to this type of problem. This is how the country's Ministry of Health (MINSAL) has decided to support telemedicine applications developed in different areas over the last few years, improving care in different pathologies [4]. Applications such as teleophthalmology, teledermatology and telecardiology are part of the portfolio of services being delivered in the public sector today to improve access and care for patients. But what is the true scope of these applications? This research can be a source of information and input for any institutions or health facilities that want to carry out intervention programs in its population with telemedicine programs.

The author of this Chapter, is an electronic engineer (Pontificia Universidad Católica de Valparaíso), with a Master's degree in Computer Engineering (Universidad Técnica Federico Santa María), and another Master's degree in Management of Health Organizations (Universidad de Valparaíso), he estimates that as an academic and researcher at the University of Valparaíso, it was necessary to generate knowledge and experiences, to know and spread the real state of telemedicine in the country. In this chapter, he appeals to his work experience acquired in the area of telemedicine, as Chief of Information Technology of a Public Health Service, and summarizes a sequence of background information resulting from his own work, projects, and research.

2. Theoretical framework

First of all, we mention that Telehealth aims to improve access and opportunity to health services, and it must be developed under the model of integrated health services networks (IHSN), defined by the Pan American Health Organization (PAHO) as "a network of organizations that provides, or arranges the provision of fair and integral health services to a defined population, and is willing to be accountable for its clinical and economic results" [5].

The Telehealth presents us with an innovative strategy that allows us to optimize specialized human resources, complementing actions and solutions that allow the benefited population to experience a substantial improvement in access to health care. This being a strategy includes the access gaps to the system and the opportunity for attention to the patients.

2.1 Telemedicine

Among the different definitions used for the term telemedicine, we can agree for its most frequent use, that is, a way of providing health services to patients who are limited to it by geography, work, or health issues. In these cases, telemedicine can improve the accessibility and efficiency of these services. In the same sense, the WHO refers to telemedicine as "the provision of health care services in cases where distance is a critical factor, carried out by health professionals who use information and communication technologies (ICTs) for the exchange of valid information to make diagnoses, prevention and treatment of diseases, ongoing training of health care professionals, as well as for research and evaluation activities, in order to improve the health of people and their communities" [4, 6].

There is a great variety of medical specialties and technological applications in telemedicine although there is no standardized categorization for the latter; they can be classified according to their applications, specialties, method of data transmission, and according to the geographical area. Regarding definitions and terminologies, it is considered necessary to standardize the following terms, from the extensive portfolio of medical specialties, which have gradually been converted into telemedicine applications. The following are some of the most representative and highly used specialties in our country [4, 7].

A. *Telecardiology:* Consists of the prevention, diagnosis, and treatment of cardiovascular diseases, especially acute myocardial infarction (AMI) at a distance. It allows the interaction of primary health care personnel (PHC) in real or deferred time and on an ambulatory basis with cardiologists to avoid geographical movement and to solve emergencies. Initially, it consisted in the interaction between the health staff and the specialist doctor (through electrocardiograms); at present, the equipment can record and send electrocardiograms, echocardiograms, heart sounds, sounds, and images.

B. *Teledermatology:* Consists in the exchange of medical information (through visual communication, or transmission of photographs or images). It allows the PHC staff to interact in real or deferred time and on an ambulatory basis with dermatologists to avoid geographical movement and grant diagnosis at a distance. Since diagnostics are mainly in images (storage/sending/receiving), it makes the consultation and subsequent response an effective way to grant consultation of diagnoses, treatments, and health care management.

C. *Teleophthalmology:* Consists of the referral of the patient, where health personnel interact with the patient and a specialist doctor, about a problem related to eye injuries. It allows deeper exploration and detection of other lesions or alterations, such as the screening of diabetic retinopathy.

D. *Telepsychiatry:* Consist of the referral between the patient and the specialist doctor, at the different levels of pathologies, such as depression, anxiety, stress, schizophrenia, use of substances, etc.; through videoconferencing interventions in adults, children and adolescents, and mental health programs.

E. *Telenephrology:* Consists of the referral between a family doctor in the deferent center, and a nephrologist (online or deferred, with or without the patient), about the history of a patient with chronic kidney disease, and his/her possible treatment and evolution.

F. *Teleneurology:* Consists of the referral and provision of neurological assistance between the patient and the specialist doctor; when they are not present in the same place and/or temporary moment (through videoconference, images or data of the clinical history).

G. *Other Teleconsultations:* Consists of the consultation or referral, between the patient, the health personnel, and a specialist doctor (in a remote location), in real time or deferred, about diagnoses, treatments, medical images, or requirements, in a certain pathology (not included in the others named before).

H. *Teleradiology:* Transmission of radiological images from one place to another for the purpose of diagnosis, interpretation or consultation. To be able to make teleradiology, a digital X-ray equipment, or a conventional X-ray machine plus a digitizer are usually required. In this case, a remote service is already provided. The interaction happens here between the X-ray technician and the doctor.

Also, within telemedicine, two basic modes of operation can be distinguished: (a) in real time or synchronous mode, (b) in deferred time or asynchronous mode, or, as it is also known, the storage-sending mode [4, 8, 9].

For the synchronous modality, it is required to schedule an appointment and simultaneous availability of the agents that will interact in the session; it is based on the interaction in real time and live, which allows live communication from the treating doctor or another professional, patient, and specialist, the latter being who will deliver diagnostic and/or therapeutic guidelines to the treating doctor. We have to distinguish two types of synchronous modality: programmed (making an appointment) and urgency (when the patient needs to talk to the doctor at that same moment).

The asynchronous modality allows the storage and transfer of data and fixed images (store and forward) in "deferred," which are sent to a specialist professional along with the patient's medical history, so the doctor issues a diagnostic and therapeutic advice. In this modality, there is no direct interaction between the specialist and the patient, and the asynchronous mode is used in those cases in which the diagnosis or consultation of the information sent does not imply an emergency situation, and its query can be deferred in minutes and hours, using, for example, the mail as a means of transmitting the information. This modality is the one that has greater volume of activity at the present time.

Telemedicine is characterized because distance exists between the sender and the receiver (doctor-patient), so it is necessary to use some means of communication to transmit the necessary information, and that at both ends, there are some means or equipment that codifies the shared information. It is also essential to have the necessary infrastructure to establish a telecommunication (teleconsultation). For this, there are indispensable elements that are used for the use of telemedicine. Among the minimum components that a telemedicine network must contain to ensure adequate medical support from a distance, we can mention [10]:

- patients;
- health personnel in primary care (PHC) or first contact (general doctor, nurse);
- the consulting center (fixed or mobile);
- medical specialists or subspecialists;
- reference centers or telediagnosis (second or third hospital level);
- an adequate telecommunication network;
- the necessary equipment (video conferencing equipment, medical peripherals); and
- company and/or technical support staff.

2.2 Latin American experiences

According to the World Health Organization (WHO) [10], telemedicine is defined as "the provision of health care services, in which distance is a critical factor, by professionals who appeal to the technologies of the information and communication in order to exchange data to make diagnoses, recommend treatments, and prevent diseases and injuries, as well as for ongoing training of health care professionals and in research and evaluation activities, in order to improve health of the people and communities in which they live."

One of the first activities carried out from the academic point of view was to investigate and learn about telemedicine experiences in the countries of Latin America. To this end, certain sources of information were used, and it could be established that although some of these publications had been published in Santiago, Chile, none of them mentioned a case of Chilean experience [11].

According to the specialized literature on the subject (only in Latin America), there are countries such as Costa Rica, Brazil, El Salvador, Ecuador, Mexico, Colombia, and Panama, where the Government has defined and established a "telemedicine policy," with precise guidelines regarding objectives, prioritization of projects, processes, and concrete actions with allocation of resources [6, 11–13].

2.3 Advantages and disadvantages

As mentioned above, ICTs offer great potential to solve the challenges faced by developed and developing countries in providing accessible, timely, and quality medical services. Telemedicine uses ICTs to overcome geographical barriers and increase access to health care services. This benefits rural areas and marginalized communities that do not have direct access to specific health care.

Telemedicine is one of the most prominent, known and used branches of Telehealth, according to the American Telemedicine Association (ATA). Telemedicine is the exchange of medical information between two actors that are not located in the same space, which can be doctor/patient, or doctor/doctor; through electronic communications, through some means of electronic communication, in order to improve the health status of a patient. It includes "a growing variety of applications and services that use videoconferencing, email, smartphones, wireless communications and other forms of telecommunications technology" [4].

The specialized literature on the subject mentions that there are several advantages and benefits that different telemedicine applications can bring [9, 10].

2.3.1 Advantages

One of the most relevant advantages of Telemedicine is the reduction of inequalities in the population to have access to health services, regardless of geographical location. It also facilitates equity in access to such services by providing high quality universal medical care.

It also provides patients with specialized medical care, in places where they do not have it (or it is very time consuming), reducing the need for travel by patients and/or health professionals.

It allows the reduction of times and waiting lists; by means of a shorter time in the realization of the diagnosis and consequently, less time in the treatment, avoiding delays in the serious cases that could cause problems for the patient.

It manages to increase the efficiency of the system by optimizing health care resources, improving demand management, reducing hospital stays, and reducing repetitions of examinations as well as medical acts.

It also allows the decentralization of demand in medical care, avoiding the saturation of emergency services, as well as in second and third level hospital units.

You can also specify benefits by groups of beneficiaries:

1. For patients: Diagnoses and faster and more timely treatments; reduction in the number of further and multiple examinations; comprehensive and continuous care from the first moment; the discomfort of displacements for patients and relatives is avoided, to consult a specialist doctor, reducing possible expenses. It also facilitates the intradomiciliary management of the disabled

patient, prostrate or unable to move; and families can stay longer and closer to the patient, and have more direct contact with health personnel.

2. For health personnel in primary care (PHC), or first contact: New possibilities to consult with specialists; the possibility of avoiding inconvenient displacements; more elements of judgment when making decisions, being able to verify diagnoses and request a second opinion with the specialists; improves the quality and timeliness of the background to be able to diagnose. It also improves the flow of information transmission, avoiding the loss (or duplication) of reports and exams; grants the possibility for training and training of health professionals, through continuing medical education.

3. For hospitals: Reduction of the risk of loss of exams and images; faster and more accurate diagnoses and treatments; better and faster communication between different services; eliminate duplicate information; more effective care equipment and services; greater economy in the expenses derived from the transportation of patients; and an optimization of internal administrative processes.

4. Advantages for the health system: Better use and use of resources (physical, human, and financial); better management of public health and the health care network; additional resources for teaching students; more flexible and timely scientific and statistical analyzes; an increase in the accessibility of information at all levels of care; and allow the establishment of medical support networks at the country level.

2.3.2 Potential drawbacks or challenges of telemedicine

Also, the introduction of telemedicine sometimes has its disadvantages, or potential drawbacks for its correct implementation. Among which:

- Less accuracy for the diagnosis of certain images transmitted with telemedicine in relation to the original images, if the ICTs are appropriate for us. There is a risk of loss of data and images (resolution) due to the compression of said data to increase the transmission speed.

- Aspects linked to security and confidentiality in the doctor-patient relationship through appropriate interfaces, with possible legal and ethical implications.

- Increase of the demand to the specialists, being able to reach not being able to satisfy the high assistance volume of patients.

- The programs used in telemedicine should be compared with other alternative options, ensuring that in addition to offering very fast services are also viable services.

- Obstacles may arise during the implementation and setting up of this new technology, by health professionals, by the typical reaction to change, fear of losing their jobs, or lack of training.

- The implementation of telemedicine systems depends on an adequate telecommunications infrastructure. And, the technology and infrastructure must be sufficiently developed to support the implementation of large-scale telemedicine; the aspects of good bandwidth and quality of service (QoS) are important.

- It is very important to have a diagnosis and survey of the real needs of the population so that the health services are not prey to the providers of equipment and services (and that they do not consider the real needs of the users). The programs used in telemedicine must be compared with other alternative options, to make sure that in addition to offering services with speed and quality, they are also viable services.

3. Status of telemedicine in Chile

3.1 Experiences and previous investigations

Health spending represents, in Chile, about 10% of GDP and grows at a rate close to 10%. This level of spending and growth is comparable to that of the OECD countries [8]. It is a known fact that if the efficiency in the use of resources is not increased, the maintenance of the system will be unsustainable, causing serious damage to the quality and life expectancy of the people. In this context, various technologies, services, and strategies have emerged in the world to empower them in order to overcome the current gaps (specialists, waiting lists, etc.) and those that are to come (chronic diseases, increasing life expectancy). Medicine currently has a development of therapeutic options greater in quantity and effectiveness than at any other time in its history. A fundamental concern lies in the ability of the health system to reach the people who require these therapies in an effective and equitable manner. The development of technologies that support clinical systems and health management provide an opportunity to shorten gaps in effective coverage that achieve the development of a fair and efficient health system.

In the case of Chile, there is a consensus on the urgent need to incorporate technologies and improvements in management. Therefore, a specialized strategic program is required to reduce gaps, catalyze and streamline regulatory processes, and the adoption of technologies and services, delivering measurable and demonstrable results in the short term that will position Chile as a leader in the region.

As previously mentioned, while several Latin American countries were advancing in telemedicine policies and plans, Chile did not appear in the specialized literature. Several initiatives and advances in this regard began to be developed. In Chile, telemedicine has been seen as a necessary solution to face the problems of coverage, shortage of specialists and care in remote areas, a problem that is especially relevant given the geography of the country. Thus, from 1993 onward, a series of public and private initiatives have been developed for the realization of telemedicine services. The development of these initiatives can be summarized in the following milestones that also mark the history of this discipline in the country.

The author of the chapter carried out an investigation to quantitatively know the specialty medical consultations based on the use of telemedicine. In Chile, given the information needs required by MINSAL (Ministry of Health), it is required that each establishment with an assigned DEIS code (recognized by the Department of Health Statistics and Information), report its production of attentions and population in control individually; to then consolidate it in the Health Service to which it belongs, and finally send it to MINSAL [7].

All the above information is consolidated in the REM (monthly statistical summary), which MINSAL receives in a timely manner from all the Health

Establishments in the country. Among them, there is REM-A07, which is used by all establishments with Medical Care of Specialties, such as: Therapeutic Diagnostic Center (CDT), Hospital Specialty Center (CAE), Health Reference Center (CRS), and Community Center for Mental Health (COSAM); and also all the PHC establishments (CESFAM) that have a specialist doctor. In particular, Section F of this summary corresponds to the provision of specialty medical consultation granted to outpatients from various primary health care centers or hospitals of low complexity, which require remote assistance from a Specialist Physician through the use of ICTs, registering the production of specialty consultations by telemedicine.

For the study, official data were requested from MINSAL, through requests for Transparency Law (public access); and the period between January 2014 and December 2016 (3 years) was included, considering that all specialties were already mature enough and in normal use. However, not all specialties have the same coverage in all regions of the country; and all the information that is delivered is available for confirmation. To date, seven categories are being registered and consolidated in the country: telecardiology, teledermatology, telepsychiatry, teleophthalmology, telenephrology, teleneurology, and other teleconsultations.

The different data were stored in a matrix repository. The global statistics of this original work are shown in the graph of **Figure 1**. With a universe of 139,763, registered care at the country level (for 36 months), correspond to 24,187 throughout 2014, to 44,906 in 2015, and 70,670 in 2016; representing a notable increase (292%) in said period. Of these, 58,281 correspond to men, and 81,482 to women. Of the total of them: 12,031 attentions for beneficiaries of less than 15 years, 62,348 of more 15 and less than 60 years; and to 65,384 for patients over 60 years of age. In **Table 1**, the medical consultations by telespecialty and age range are shown, and its graph is shown in **Figure 2**.

Figure 3 shows teleconsultation total by specialty (during the 36 months of study). In **Figure 4**, the evolution of the specialties during the 3-year investigation is shown.

According to the study, of the seven specialties, the largest medical consultations correspond to teledermatology (26.8%), teleophthalmology (24.7%), and telecardiology (22.1%) and those with the least registration are the telepsychiatry specialties (1, 5%), teleneurology (1.8%), and telenephrology (2.6%).

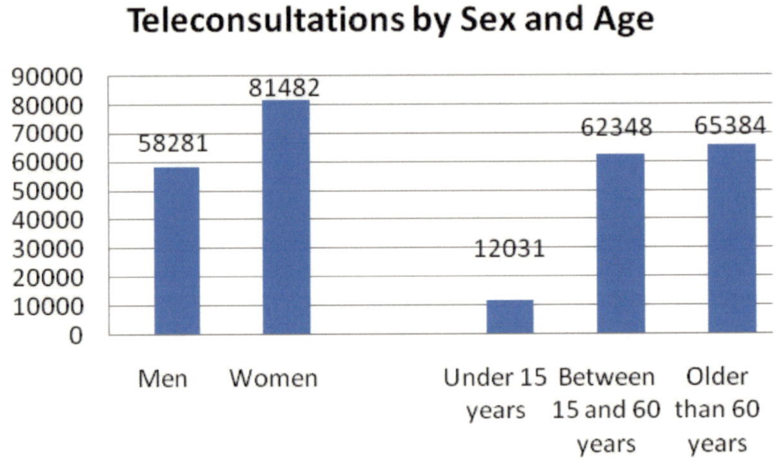

Figure 1.
Teleconsultations by sex and age (2014–2016).

Specialties	<15 years	15< years <60	>60 years
Telecardiology	419	16,022	14,486
Teledermatology	8992	17,932	10,500
Telepsychiatry	684	1076	288
Teleophthalmology	32	15,210	19,251
Telenephrology	18	837	2813
Teleneurology	455	1163	887
Other teleconsultations	1431	10,108	17,159
Total	12,031	62,348	65,384

Table 1.
Specialties by age range (2014–2016).

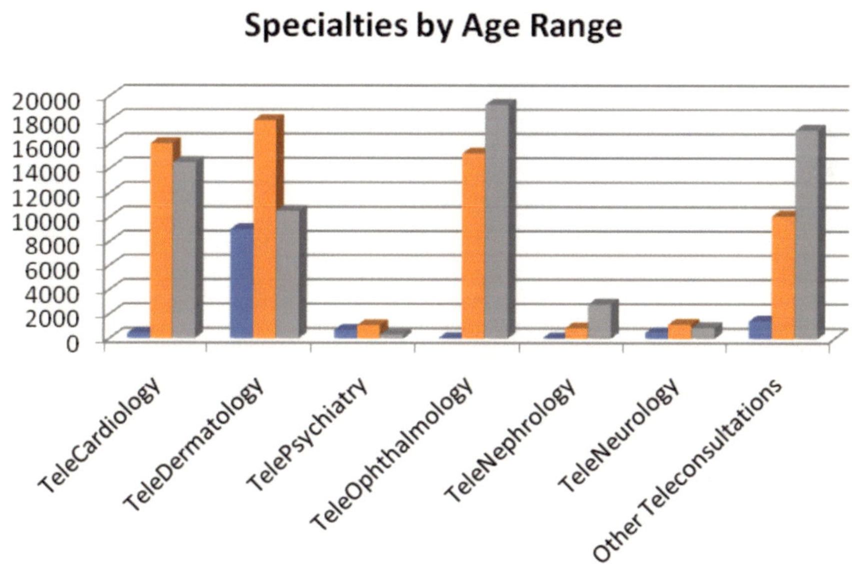

Figure 2.
Specialties by age range (2014–2016).

3.2 Projects and programs

As mentioned, currently, Chile does not have a directory that allows the possibility of publicizing and sharing the different experiences in telemedicine that have been carried out or are being carried out, either in the form of pilot plans, projects or stable programs. Based on the report "National Telehealth Program," and as another contribution by the author, the information was organized into categories according to the type of telemedical service that is delivered, and the direction of the flow of information was also defined, defining the derivative centers (who requests) and the centers of reference (who answers), indicating the telespecialty that is offered.

The records were grouped into three cases:

- Projects, which are cases in which different health facilities, by initiative and own funds, establish an agreement with a specialty reference center, and perform types of care according to the specialty they require, see **Table 2**.

- The National Strategic Programs, which are initiatives and actions initiated by the MINSAL and which establishes and finances the start-up of care in almost all health facilities in the country, is shown in **Table 3**.

- The Telemedicine Platforms and Committees are the telemedicine services provided by several specialized companies in this type of service, or Centers specialized in Telemedicine, see **Table 4**.

3.3 Legislative framework

In Chile, there is no specific legislation on Telehealth and/or Telemedicine, however, reference is made to International documents that propose the adoption and execution, by the Member States, of telehealth policies or e-health, as a strategy

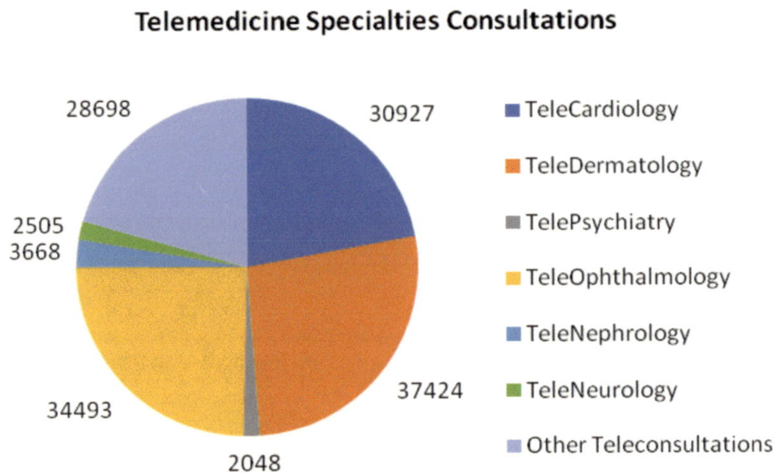

Figure 3.
Teleconsultations by specialties (2014–2016).

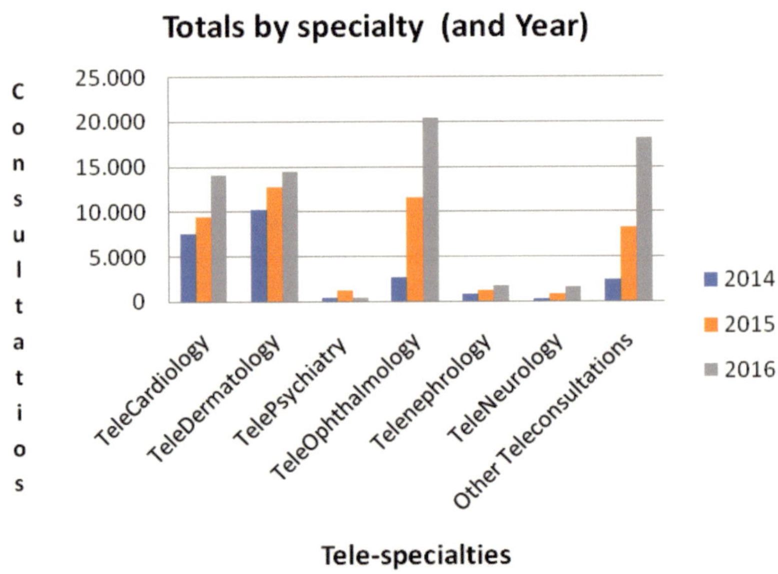

Figure 4.
Evolution of the telespecialties by year.

Year Start	Derivative Center	Reference Center	Classification	Project Specialty
1993	Universidad Católica	Dr. Sotero del Rio Hospital	Telediagnosis	Comparison of traditional diagnosis vs telediagnosis
			Telecapacitation	Development of optimal methods of remote collaboration
1995	Clinica Alemana Temuco	Clinica Alemana Santiago	Telediagnosis	Teleradiology
1998	Juan Fernández Island	Clinica las Condes	Telediagnosis	Telediagnosis
2000	UCH Clinical Hospital	Js. Johns Hospital (EE. UU.)	Telecapacitation	Telecapacitation
2001	Carlos Van Buren Hospital	Universidad de Valparaiso	Telecapacitation	Transmisión de imágenes neuroquirúrgicas
2003	Antártica	UCH Clinical Hospital	Telemonitoring	Teleradiology
2009	San Carlos Hospital Linares Hospital Angol Hospital	Las Higueras Hospital	Telediagnosis	Telecardiology Telepsychiatry
2012	Queilén Hospital Achao Hospital	Castro Hospital	Teleconsultations	Teledermatology
2012	Puerto Natales Hospital Puerto Williams Hospital Porvenir Hospital	Clinical Hospital Magallanes	Teleconsultations	Telecardiology Teledermatology Teleradiology
2013	La Calera Hospital La Ligua Hospital Petorca Hospital Limache Hospital Quintero Hospital	Gustavo Fricke Hospital	Teleconsultations Tele informes Telediagnosis	Telecardiology Teleradiology
2015	El Pino Hospital	Universidad de Santiago	Telediagnosis	Teledermatology
2015	Iquique Teletón	Santiago Teletón	Teleconsultations Telediagnosis	Telerehabilitation
2016	UPC de Hospital Regional de Coyhaique	Hospital del Tórax	Telediagnosis Telecare	Teleurology Teletraumatology Telepsychiatry Teleneurology
2017	Los Ángeles PHC Centers	Concepción Teletón	Teleconsultations Telediagnosis	Telerehabilitation
2017	Quillota Hospital La Serena Hospital San Felipe Hospital Antofagasta Hospital	Gustavo Fricke Hospital + Hospital Carlos Van Buren Hospital	Teleconsultations	Telecardiology
2017	Molina Hospital Curepto Hospital Constitución Hospital Hualañé Hospital Chanco Hospital Licantén Hospital Longaví Commune CESFAM	El Maule Health Service	Telediagnosis Telemonitoring	Telepsychiatry
2017	Sename	CIMT + UCH Clinical Hospital	Teleconsultations	Telepsychiatry
2018	San Martin Hospital	Barros Luco Hospital	Telemonitoring Telediagnosis	Tele Trombólisis or Tele ACV
2018	San Martin Hospital Quilpué Hospital	Gustavo Fricke Hospital	Telediagnosis Teleconsultations	Attention of specialists and subspecialists
2018	Magallanes Hospital	UCH Clinical Hospital	Telecare Teleconsultations	Telerehabilitation Telepsychiatry Telegenetics
2018	CESFAM Semilleros CESFAM Paulina Avendaño, Talcahuano CESFAM San Vicente, Talcahuano CESFAM Los Cerros, Talcahuano CESFAM Hualpencillo de Hualpen, Comuna de Tomé CESFAM Alberto Reyes, Comuna de Tomé	Las Higueras Hospital	Telediagnosis Teleconsultations Telemonitoring	Teleneurology

Table 2.
Main telemedicine projects.

to improve health of those States. In this regard, the World Health Organization, in 2005 agreed Resolution WHA.58.28, adopted at the 58th World Health Assembly, which indicates that there was awareness that advances in information and

Year Start	Derivative Center	Reference Center	Classification	Program Specialty
2009	29 Health Services	Dermatology Center	Teleconsultations	Teledermatology
2012	Hospitals of low complexity and PHC	28 Health Services	Teleconsultations Telecapacitation	Contact of specialists of hospitals of medium / high complexity with doctors in training in hospitals of low complexity or PHC
2014	María Pinto, Alhué y Curacaví Centers	San José de Melipilla Hospital	Teleconsultations	Teleconsultations in patients who require anticoagulant treatment
		Peñaflor Hospital		
		San Juan de Dios Hospital		
	Curacaví Hospital	San Juan de Dios Hospital		
	Isla de Maipo y El Monte Communes	Talagante Hospital		
2014	PHC Centers	San Borja Arriaran Hospital, Metropolitano Central Health Service	Telereports	Child Neuropsychiatry
2016	El Pino Hospital	Metropolitano Sur Health Service	Teleconsultations	Telecardiology
	Talagante Hospital			
	Copiapó Hospital			
2016	Rancagua Hospital	Tórax Hospital	Telemonitoring	Telemedicine for Extracorporeal Oxygenation Therapy
	San Fernando Hospital			
	Coyhaique Hospital			
	Castro Hospital			
	San Camilo Hospital			
	Padre Hurtado Hospital	Sotero Del Rio Hospital		
	La Florida Hospital			
	Gustavo Fricke Hospital			
	Quillota Hospital			
	Quilpué Hospital			
	Carlos Van Buren Hospital			
	El Pino Hospital			
	Complejo Asistencial Barros Luco			
2017	Copiapó Hospital	Carlos Van Buren Hospital	Teleconsultations	Neuro Surgical Telemedicine Network
	Vallenar Hospital			
	La Serena Hospital			
	Gustavo Fricke Hospital			
	San Camilo Hospital			
	Los Andes Hospital			
2017	Arica Health Service	Roberto del Rio Hospital, Metropolitano Norte Health Service	Teleconsultations	Telemedicine in Network of Operable Congenital Heart Diseases
	Atacama Health Service			
	Coquimbo Health Service			
	Valparaiso-San Antonio Health Service			
	Metropolitano Central Health Service			
	Servicio de Salud Metropolitano Sur			
	O'Higgins Health Service			
2017	29 Health Services	Public Assistance Hospital, Metropolitano Central Health Service	Teleconsultations Telereports	Telemedicine in a network of serious burns

Table 3.
Main National Telemedicine Programs.

communication technologies have generated expectations regarding health; and recalling resolution WHA51.9, he emphasized that e-health consists of the support that the cost-effective and safe use of information and communication technologies offers to health and related fields, including health services, health care, health surveillance and documentation, as well as health education, knowledge, and research [4], and urged the Member States to develop and promote a range of activities, including the establishment of national networks and centers of excellence working on e-health, and in particular on exemplary practices, policy coordination, and technical support for the delivery of health care, improvement of services,

Year Start	Derivative Center	Reference Center	Classification	Program Specialty
2005	Emergency Primary Care Services (all the country)	Report Central	Telereports	Telecardiology
2005	General Access	Salud Responde	Telecapacitation	Teleconsultations
			Teleassistant	
2009	29 Health Services		Teleconsultations	Teledermatology
2012	Talcahuano Health Service	Cardiovascular Health Program	Telereports	Telenephrology
	Concepción Health Service			
	Arauco Health Service			
	Ñuble Health Service			
	O'Higgins Health Service			
	Metropolitano Sur Oriente Health Service			
	Metropolitano Norte Health Service			
	Reloncaví Health Service			
	Metropolitano Occidente Health Service			
2013	124 Ophthalmological Primary Care Unit	Teleophthalmology Platform	Telereports	Teleophthalmology
2016	Specialty Centers of the country	VIH Network (Lucio Córdova Hospital)	Telerehabilitation and teletreatment	Telemedicine VIH Net
2017	San José Hospital, SSMN	RIS/PACS Platform	Telereports	Teleradiology
	Roberto del Río Hospital, SSMN		Telediagnosis	Teleimaging
	Instituto Nacional del Cáncer, SSMN			
2017	Dr. Juan Noé Crevani Hospital	Cardiological Committee on Congenital Heart Diseases Operable by Telemedicine (Metropolitano Norte Health Service, and Cardiological Equipment of the Roberto del Río Children's Hospital) - SSMN	Telediagnosis	Telecardiology
	Copiapó Hospital			
	La Serena Hospital		Teleconsultations	
	Carlos Van Buren Hospital			
	El Carmen Hospital		Telemonitoring	
	El Pino Hospital			
	Dr. Exequiel González Cortés Hospital			
	Barros Luco Trudeau Hospital			
	Rancagua Hospital			
2018	Concepción Hospital	Oncology and Radiotherapy Center	Telerehabilitation	Teleradiology
	Herminda Martin Hospital		Telediagnosis	

Table 4.
Main platforms based on telemedicine.

information to the citizen, development of means of action and surveillance. In relation to the legal norms that allow and sustain the development of the Telehealth Program, we can mention as the first foundation the Political Constitution of Chile, in its Article 19, numeral 9, this ensures all the people the right to health protection and establishes as a duty of the State to protect free and equal access to actions for the promotion, protection and recovery of health and rehabilitation of the individual.

On the other hand [4], Article 3 of Law No. 18.575, Constitutional Organic General Bases of the State Administration states that: "The State Administration is at the service of the human person; Its purpose is to promote the common good by attending to public needs in a continuous and permanent manner and promoting the development of the country through the exercise of the powers conferred by the Constitution and the Law, and the approval, execution and control of Policies, Plans, Programs and Actions of national, regional and communal scope."

The aforementioned standards constitute an obligation for the State and that is why actions must be taken to ensure access to health care, whether these actions are carried out in a conventional manner or whether new strategies should be implemented.

In addition, Article 1, DFL N°1, of 2005, of MINSAL, which establishes a consolidated, coordinated, and systematized text of Decree Law No. 2763 of 1979 and of Law Nos. 18,933 and 18,469 reinforces the provisions of the Political Constitution and establishes the responsibility of the Ministry of Health to guarantee such right, as well as to coordinate, control, and when appropriate, execute such actions. According to the above, in our country telehealth strategies will be implemented within the framework of current regulations and associated with defined clinical-care processes, complying with the standards of face-to-face care [4].

In relation to the applicability of the telemedicine modality in the health benefits associated with the Auge-GES and non-GES Plans (pathologies with and without guarantees), and regarding the legal medical liability associated with this benefit, the Legal Division of MINSAL has informed, through Memorandums A15 N°04995, of December 31, 2013 and Memorandum A 15 N°0223, of September 3, 2015, as follows: "Under the modality of telemedicine it is possible to incorporate that set of medical assistance procedures that are materially executed remotely, using different means of communication and image technologies, in order to collaborate in the care of health and ranging from clinical background and examinations to technical assistance in medical work of any kind, such as invasive and non-invasive procedures, which are developed remotely and under specific professional supervision." Also, "Telemedicine is part of collaborative professional procedures that contribute to the health care of people and that is linked to other procedures and professional and technical actions performed by professionals, technicians, and administrative staff in health. In this case, the work of assistance developed by telemedicine by an ad-hoc professional, as the case may be, is delivered to a health team responsible for the face-to-face care of a person, for the formulation of due care that includes diagnosis and treatment of the case."

In addition, it is contemplated that [4, 14]:

1. Law No. 20,584, which regulates the rights and duties of people in relation to actions related to their health care, establishes with respect to informed consent, in Article 14, that this is required for all health care and it will generally be done verbally. Notwithstanding the foregoing, the patient's consent must be recorded in writing in the case of "surgical interventions, invasive diagnostic, and therapeutic procedures and, in general, for the application of procedures that involve a relevant and known risk to the health of the affected person."

2. Telemedicine care in Specialty Consultation whether Ambulatory, Hospitalization or Urgency, is not an invasive procedure or that involves significant risk to health. Nor are the reports of procedures or examinations carried out by telemedicine. In this context, it is not necessary to have a signed record of such consent, it being understood that, in the act of medical care, the professional explains to the patient the process of care to be developed through telemedicine and the continuity of care associated with it. In addition to the above, it must be considered that the benefits to be developed by telemedicine must be defined in the Portfolio of Establishment Services and Derivation Map, which must be informed to the Community. The Information and Communication Technologies (ICTs) to be

used as support for telemedicine services must comply with the Information Security issued by MINSAL and with the provisions of Law No. 20,584 that regulates the rights and duties of people in relation to actions linked to their health care and Law No. 19,628 on the protection of privacy. At this point, mention that if the established is fulfilled, a written record of informed consent is neither required to take photographs in the context of medical care, nor to record a telemedicine care performed by the MINSAL Videoconference Network, in a context of critical care or of urgency and that it is required to support for possible future audits. In that sense, article 5, letter (c) of the aforementioned Law No. 20,584, states in relation to the right to a dignified treatment, that providers must "Respect and protect the privacy and honor of the person during their health care. In particular, these rights must be ensured in relation to the taking of photographs, recordings or films, whatever their purpose or use. In any case, for the taking of photographs, recordings or filming for journalistic or advertising purposes or uses, written authorization from the patient or his legal representative will be required." In this way, it is possible to conclude that those recordings or taking photographs for purposes other than journalistic or advertising, do not require the express authorization of the patient, however, the protection of their rights.

It also details several important ethical aspects that should be considered for telemedicine care [4].

4. National program

4.1 Objectives

As mentioned previously, while several Latin American countries developed policies and programs in telemedicine, others did not. The CORFO (Production Development Corporation) created, from April 2015, a Strategic Program "Health + Development," whose main objective was to strengthen the environment for the development of the services, technologies, and health management industry; and ways to effectively contribute to improve the national health system and the quality of life of patients [8]. The program aims to generate sectors capable of producing new goods and services, develop industries, and generate poles of innovation. Then the National Telemedicine Day was held in the city of Valdivia (July 2015) [15]. And in order to continue advancing in the area, it was created in conjunction with the National University Network (REUNA), a working group composed of representatives of different universities, CORFO, Ministry of Health, FONASA, CEPAL, REUNA, and RUTE (University Network of Telemedicine, Brazil), where the advances in the area of telemedicine were discussed and the main challenges that needed to be addressed for its growth.

There was a collective consensus on the need to have a telemedicine policy, which finally progressed toward a National Telemedicine Program, which provides a conceptual framework and technical, strategic, administrative, organizational, and financial guidelines for the development and optimal functioning of the strategies of telemedicine that are already installed in the Health Networks of Chile.

As part of the Strategic Health and Development Program, the Ministry of Economy, Development, and Tourism requested the RAND Health Corporation to create a roadmap to guide the development of information technology (ICT) in health in the public health system in Chile. This project had two phases. For the first phase of this project, the current status of the adoption and implementation of ICT in health in Chile is described. For the second phase, a roadmap was designed that focuses on key objectives and activities designed to foster growth in the adoption and successful implementation of health ICTs in the public sector in Chile, including telemedicine [16, 17].

If we focus on the competitive advantages, in terms of clinical and hospital services (public and private), Chile is next to Brazil, a leader in the region. In terms of connectivity, another crucial element to develop this type of industry, the country ranks 35 out of 144 according to the ranking of the World Economic Forum (WEF) [8]. Just to compare, Colombia ranks 63rd in the ranking, Brazil ranks 69th and Mexico 79th in the same ranking [1, 2]. Finally, Chile has been a pioneer in the implementation of fiber optic connections for the transfer of complex and high-speed information, highlighting in particular the effort made by the National University Network (REUNA) and the austral cable project currently under study. On the demand side, the main driver for the development of this program, we find a health sector where public and private spending increases steadily as a consequence of factors such as the aging of the population, the increase of chronic diseases and the growing lack of specialists. Only by way of example, spending on health in the public sector has increased only 11, 8% in the last year, reaching almost 8% of GDP as reported by the Government's Budget Office.

Based on what was stated in point 3, for the current development of Telehealth it was required to address in a Program [4], the following areas:

- Decrease of access barriers, improving the opportunity and continuity in the attention of the user population, for the satisfaction of their health needs.

- It will allow to diminish the impact of the deficit of specialists in areas that present gaps in the country.

- It will allow the optimization of existing resources in the Network, positively impacting the pocket expense15 of the population.

- It will favor the technical transfer from the health teams between the different levels of care, facilitating training, and continuing education. Also, the interrelation between professionals for the promotion of good professional practices.

- It will allow to define the technical competences of the human resource, its functions and profile according to the actions to be developed in the different components of the program.

- Having organizational definitions of the program will facilitate its development and implementation in places where it is not yet installed. By defining its organizational aspects will allow the program to develop and maintain in time independent of the political changes that occur in the country.

- It will allow improving communications coverage, connectivity, and its quality, and the equipment required for telemedicine actions.

- It will help to clarify the legal, ethical, and regulatory framework existing in Chile, for the application of telemedicine and will lay the foundations for a future technical standard.

- By defining its organizational aspects will allow the program to develop and maintain in time independent of the political changes that occur in the country.

- It will favor the interrelation between professionals for the promotion of good professional practices.

This Program defines Telehealth in Chile as: a strategy based on the Model of Comprehensive Care of Family and Community Health [4], in the context of Integrated Health Services Networks [4], and that through the use of technology information and communications, facilitates the provision of distance services from the field of promotion, prevention, diagnosis, treatment, rehabilitation, and palliative care, focused on the person in their socio-cultural context and throughout their life course, with the purpose of maintain an optimal state of health and continuity of care for the population, thus improving equity in access, exercise of rights, opportunity, and quality of care through its three components: tele-education, telemedicine, and telecare.

The general objective of the Program is: to generate the technical, technological, administrative, organizational, and financial conditions to develop the three components of Telehealth in the Health Services, and in this way contribute to improving access and equity in people's integral health, and the fulfillment of the health objectives of the decade 2011–2020. The principles, specific objectives, and associated characteristics are detailed in the Program itself.

4.2 Lines of action

The lines of action of the Telehealth program in Chile are based on three components [4], as shown in **Figure 5**.

4.2.1 Tele-education

The general objective is to provide a form of continuous learning, applied to educational processes that integrate the various components and actors, through the use of Information and Communication Technologies, favoring the transfer or generation of knowledge without restrictions of space, time, or distance. It is a planned training and learning process, developed with the support of Information and Communication Technologies, aimed at both the internal and external user and the community, within the framework of a flexible process in time, space, and form, facilitating this accessibility to the formative meeting.

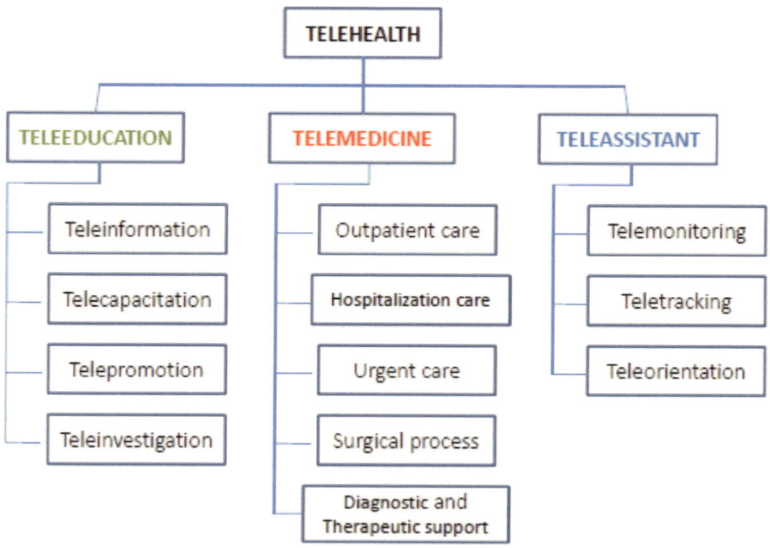

Figure 5.
Lines of Action Nation Program.

4.2.2 Telemedicine

The general objective is to grant attention and care with the use of telemedicine strategies for the delivery of medical and non-medical remote health services with timely access and quality standards to health care that also reinforces networking, establishing permanent links that ensure the continuity of people's attention. The areas of application of telemedicine correspond to the following Processes: Open Care Process: Primary Health Care; Ambulatory Specialties Care; Attention Process in Hospitalization: Hospitalization Care; Emergency Care Process: Attention in PHC and Hospital Emergency Unit; Surgical Process: Major Ambulatory Surgery-Surgery of Greater Complexity; Diagnostic and Therapeutic Support Process: Procedures, Exams, Analysis samples.

4.2.3 Teleassistant (or Telecare)

Its objective is to allow people to connect with the health network, coordinating the available resources and devices. Involves direct and bidirectional actions, between a person outside a health facility and a team and/or an application, which interact through health information and communication technologies (TIC) for the maintenance, control and improvement of individual health. It has three areas of action: Telemonitoring, Teletracking, and Teleorientation.

5. Conclusion

In this chapter, I wanted to enumerate the different experiences related to telemedicine in Chile, the advancement, the main characteristics, and expectations of the National Program of Telemedicine. I summarized the main concepts involved and the advantages, disadvantages, and challenges that this discipline faces. I have included some research done by me as a contribution to the development of the telemedicine in the future. It is a first version which can be supplemented and improved later.

Conflict of interest

The author declares that he does not have any conflict of interest.

Author details

Antonio Rienzo Renato
School of Biomedical Engineering, Universidad de Valparaíso, Chile

*Address all correspondence to: antonio.rienzo@uv.cl

References

[1] Naciones Unidas. Envejecimiento. 2018. Available from: http://www.un.org/es/sections/issues-depth/ageing/index.html

[2] OMS. Envejecimiento y Salud; Notas Descriptivas. 5 de Febrero del 2018. Available from: http://www.who.int/es/news-room/fact-sheets/detail/envejecimiento-y-salud

[3] Herrera A. Telemedicina: Una herramienta poco explotada. Revista Obstetricia y Ginecología. Hospital Santiago Oriente. 2006;**1**(3): 233-236. Available from: http://www.revistaobgin.cl/files/pdf/articulosde_revision_233a2360.pdf

[4] MINSAL. Programa Nacional de Telesalud. Subsecretaría de Redes Asistenciales; 2017. Available from: https://biblioteca.digital.gob.cl/handle/123456789/3635

[5] Staff PAHO. Redes Integradas de Servicios de Salud. Washington: Pan American Health Organization; 2010. ISBN: 978-92-75-33116-3

[6] Staff OPS/OMS. Capítulo Telemedicina; In: Conversaciones sobre eSalud. Departamento de Gestión del Conocimiento, Bioética e Investigación; Washington: EE.UU.; 2014. pp. 99. Available from: https://docplayer.es/8020140-Conversaciones-sobre-esalud.html

[7] Rienzo A. Analysis and repository of services telemedicine in Chile (2014-2015). In: 2016 IEEE International Conference on Automatica (ICA-ACCA); Curicó, Chile; October 2016. DOI: 10.1109/ICA-ACCA.2016.7778414. Available from: https://ieeexplore.ieee.org/document/7778414

[8] Staff. Informe de Mesa de Trabajo de Telemedicina. Programa Estratégico "Salud-Desarrollo"; Subsecretaría de Redes Asistenciales; 2016

[9] Rabanales J, Párraga I, et al. Tecnologías de la Información y las Comunicaciones. Telemedicina. Artículo Especial, Revista Clínica Medica Familiar;**4**(1):42-48

[10] Staff. Telemedicina; Serie Tecnologías en Salud. Volumen 3. 2da Edición. México: Centro Nacional de Excelencia Tecnológica en Salud (CENETEC). 2011. ISBN: 978-607-460-244-9. Available from: http://www.cenetec.salud.gob.mx/descargas/telemedicina/publicaciones/Volumen32daEdicion.pdf

[11] Staff CEPAL. Desarrollo de la Telesalud en América Latina. Santiago de Chile: Comisión Económica para América Latina y el Caribe (CEPAL); 2013

[12] Salazar A, Kopec A. Aplicaciones de Telecomunicaciones en Salud en la Subregión Andina. Segunda ed. Colombia: ORAS-CONHU; 2006. pp. 97-99

[13] Chueke D. Panorama de la Telemedicina en América Latina. España: Publicaciones de la Asociación Iberoamericana de Telesalud y Telemedicina; 2015

[14] MINSAL. Ordinario 2C N°247 del 29.01.2018 de la Subsecretaría de Redes Asistenciales. Santiago, Chile: Ministerio de Salud; 2018

[15] Staff. I Jornadas Nacional de Telemedicina. Valdivia: Valdivia Health Service; 2015. Available from: http://www.diariofutrono.cl/noticia/salud/2015/06/primera-jornada-nacional-de-telemedicina-se-realizara-en-valdivia

[16] RAND. Developing a Strategic Program for Chilean Health Information

Technology; Research Report. California: RAND Health Corporation; 2016. Available from: https://www.rand.org/pubs/research_reports/RR1358z1.html

[17] RAND. A Roadmap for the Development of Health Information Technology in Chile; Research Report. California: RAND Health Corporation; 2016. Available from https://www.rand.org/pubs/research_reports/RR1358z2.html

Chapter 3

Barriers to Development of Telemedicine in Developing Countries

Surya Bali

Abstract

Affordability, accessibility, availability, and quality of healthcare services have always been a burning issue for the mankind. The issue of health care is always crucial for the governments and countries irrespective of their financial status. Continuous efforts are being made by policy makers, administrators, and researchers to provide quality health care to the people at the cost that they can afford. Developed countries have adopted many alternative tools and technologies to leverage the supply of good health care but quality and cost of health care are still big issues in these countries. Developing countries are far behind in adopting technology to reduce the cost and improve the quality of health care. Telemedicine has emerged as a new hope to remove the bottlenecks in the healthcare seeking. Developing countries have adopted telemedicine technology in a hurry without proper planning and strategy. Despite more than two decades of adapting telemedicine, developing countries have not achieved any significant success in reducing the cost of care or improving the access of care. This chapter has tried to explore the various barriers to the development of telemedicine in developing countries. Proper enlisting and detailing of these barriers will definitely help governments to understand the loopholes and bottlenecks in the implementation of telemedicine and help them to develop appropriate solution.

Keywords: telehealth, telemedicine, barriers, developing countries, health care

1. Introduction

Increasing population in the developing countries has created more demand of health care. Demand of affordable and quality health care is increasing day by day. Rapid demand at the global level for healthcare management is increasing over the past few decades, increasing emphasis on healthcare quality [1]. People in poor countries have less access of health care and poor have even less access of healthcare services within the country [2]. Assessing the appropriate health care and improving the quality of care have been a serious issue in developing countries [3]. Many times, quality of public health care in developing countries has been neglected and attention is only given to technical aspects than the interpersonal components [4]. The cost of health care in developing countries has always been a crucial issue. Out of pocket expenditure on health care has increased many folds. Catastrophic health expenditure is posing a threat toward a household's financial ability to maintain its basic needs [5].

There are many barriers like geographical access, availability, affordability, and acceptability to access the health care in developing countries [6]. These barriers become more problematic to women, children, old, and physically handicapped population. Even though the health service provision and the geographical access have improved, local women may not use the services unless the provided services meet their demands in quality and cultural manners [7].

To overcome the barriers, healthcare sector is now using telemedicine solutions to increase the reach of its services to population. The mindboggling developments in Information and Communication Technologies (ICT), particularly, the web-based technologies have opened up new possibilities in providing better health care to population. Telemedicine is gradually coming up as a viable policy option for the governments in developing countries [8].

Telemedicine is the use of electronic communications and information technologies to provide clinical services when participants are at different locations [9]. Telehealth is used to encompass a broader application of technologies to distance education, health promotion, preventive services, consumer outreach, and other applications wherein electronic communications and information technologies are used to support healthcare services. According to WHO, "Telehealth involves the use of telecommunications and virtual technology to deliver health care outside of traditional healthcare facilities" [10].

In a broader and detailed way, World Health Organization (WHO) defines telehealth as: "The delivery of healthcare services, where distance is a critical factor, by all healthcare professionals using information and communication technologies for the exchange of valid information for diagnosis, treatment, and prevention of disease and injuries, research and evaluation, and for the continuing education of healthcare providers, all in the interests of advancing the health of individuals and their communities" [11].

Telemedicine is restricted to the use of IT for treatment and medical care whereas telehealth cover a broader area, where IT is used to enable the environment where people can enjoy their life at fullest. Although both these terms carry a different meaning altogether but in developing countries, both these terms are used interchangeably.

Mobile Health (mHealth) helps in patient education, health promotion, disease self-management, decrease in healthcare costs, and remote monitoring of patients and can improve healthcare delivery for developing countries [12, 13].

Lots of efforts are being made by governments (policy makers, researchers, and administrators) to develop the telemedicine network across their geographical boundaries but pace of development is slow and acceptance of technology to population is not picking up. Unfortunately, the technology that has been developed to remove or minimize the barriers to the healthcare seeking currently faces lots of barriers itself and its development has not been happening as it was expected by policy makers and researchers.

It was expected that telemedicine will reduce the burden of hospitals, suffering of patients, out of pocket expenditure, need of transport, hospital fear, and save the time and money of general public. It was also expected that it will increase the quality of care and will develop the trust among patients toward telehealthcare system. We cannot deny the partial development of telemedicine and few success stories in many parts of the world but the leverage, which we have expected from telemedicine is still lacking. Then question arises where is the problem? Why telemedicine is not picking the pace and why it is not becoming popular among service providers as well among the patients.

Many telemedicine pilot programs have been launched in developing countries in last three decades. Many evaluation studies [14, 15] have been conducted to know the success and failure of telemedicine networks and programs across the globe. Whatever success we see mostly happened in the developed countries but in most of the developing countries, success of telemedicine program is limited. This chapter will explore the various hurdles in the development of telemedicine and its operations in developing countries. Despite many benefits offered by the telemedicine, it has not been utilized fully to serve humanity and is underused [6, 7, 16–18].

There are many barriers in the adoption of telemedicine and adoption failure is serious issue, which needs to be discussed and explored. According to a study, about 75% of the telemedicine projects are abandoned or failed outright and called as failed projects and this percentage goes up to 90% in developing countries [19]. Until we are not able to find out, enlist, analyze, and understand the barriers in the deployment and development of telemedicine, we cannot ensure success of telemedicine program. Following crucial barriers are currently working in the field of telemedicine implantation and operation.

1.1 Barriers to telemedicine programs

1.1.1 Policy barriers

For smooth functioning and development of any system, we need to have definite policies and procedures at State and National level. These defined rules, regulations, procedures, and protocols are necessary to help a telemedicine system to run smoothly and safely and ensure that population receive a quality healthcare services. In many developing countries, there are no uniform and standard telemedicine policy, which leads confusion for designing telemedicine-related services, program, and its smooth implementation.

Many practitioners have fear of malpractice-related legal issues and which prevents them to actively participate and develop telemedicine program. Malpractice liability is an important barrier in the practice of telemedicine services. Certification and credential barriers also de-motivate practitioners. There is no public policy related to telemedicine for the end users, which can ensure privacy, confidentiality, and security of patient's health information during teleconsultation [8]. There are weak regulatory frameworks related to reimbursement in government as well as in private sectors against the teleconsultation services.

Because health is a state matter, state government should frame policies, programs, guidelines, and regulations regarding telemedicine practices and also allocate sufficient financial resources for telemedicine development. In few developing countries, telemedicine policy exists but implantation framework is absent [8].

There is lack of established international framework on telemedicine and also there is little consensus or understanding on uniform international standards for telemedicine practices. Telemedicine provides services across the state, country, and international borders, so there should be, at least, common international understanding on this issue.

Standardization of both hardware and software, as well as guidelines for practice, would help program managers to overcome interoperability, portability, and security issues [11].

1.1.2 Organizational structure

Lack of formal organizational structure to deliver telemedicine services is the biggest barrier for the development of telemedicine services in any country. Because being a hybrid discipline, it needs collaboration with all possible stakeholders at each level of the healthcare delivery system. Lack of collaboration between the stakeholders in the absence of specific policy becomes bottleneck in the development of telemedicine.

Department of Health and Family Welfare and Department of Information Technology should have a national level formal collaboration to develop a national telemedicine network. There are examples of such collaboration and presence of telemedicine department in few developing countries like India but it is patchy, broken, and not well established [8].

The absence of structured organization is another barrier in transforming telemedicine-related vision and political will into policies at central level. If there is no such policy, then framing of program related to accomplish those political wills become impossible. Lack of specific time bound and result-oriented programs become difficult to implement and evaluate. Systematic planning of implementation of such telemedicine programs, its concurrent monitoring, and final evaluation demands lots of trained human resources.

1.2 Lack of accreditation or regulatory bodies

There is no specificity and standardization in the practice of telemedicine, which poses accreditation issue. Lack of accreditation of telemedicine facilities creates fear among the users as well as providers. Absence of accreditation councils and regulatory bodies leaves telemedicine in isolation. Medical Councils and other health councils should take responsibility to regulate the practice and procedures of telemedicine.

There is lack of uniformity in telemedicine regulations across the world. In the absence of definite regulatory policy and guidelines, physician has apprehension and fear to practice telemedicine. Medical and health councils of different countries still find that proposed definition of telemedicine has deficiencies. These councils do not consider telemedicine as a new discipline or a new branch of medicine. Regulators consider that telemedicine presents challenges and assume that it is new and unproven. There is no clarity what to be regulated. An enabling regulatory environment is required to ensure appropriate, adequate, and quality delivery of healthcare services [20].

1.2.1 Lack of team of champions

Once telemedicine system is deployed and is placed, then there is a need of project champions, who will implement the telemedicine program. The three major champions are clinical champion, IT champion, and telemedicine champion [21]. Success of any telemedicine program depends on these champions but these champions are very few in developing countries, so most of the deployed telemedicine program die very soon after their piloting. There are also deficiencies in the training and job orientation of these champions. In most of the cases, they are not well oriented about their roles and responsibilities.

1.3 Lack of telemedicine champions

There is a paucity of dedicated, focused, and visionary telemedicine leaders in developing countries. These leaders are brand ambassadors of telemedicine and are carrying the flag of telemedicine high even in the adverse situations. Whatever telemedicine work, we see in these developing countries, are only due to individual efforts of these telemedicine champions.

1.4 Lack of clinical champions: physicians

Training is an import part of skill development and the organizations should develop a training schedule to train health professionals for smooth delivery of telemedicine services [21]. It is very important to provide training to all government officers regularly. Without proper knowledge of IT of government officers, e-governance project will never see the real face of the project [22].

Most of doctors are not aware about the latest information technology and find difficulty to used modern IT gadgets. There is lack of telemedicine experts in healthcare sectors. There is a need to include few chapters related to telemedicine in Medical education curriculum to sensitize and orient budding doctors to learn the technical part of this discipline. There should be separate telemedicine education secretariat and directorate in Ministry Medical Education like in Ministry of Health care, which will promote the development of telemedicine [8].

1.5 Lack of paraclinical champions: nurse providers

Telemedicine health services are also assisted or provided by nursing staff but their contribution in telemedicine is not recognized and acknowledged. Role of nursing staff in expansion of telemedicine could be very vital if proper training and guidance is provided to them. Most of the developing countries do not have trained telenursing officers or staff who can contribute in the development of telemedicine network.

There is also lack of proper institutional training program in the course curriculum like traditional nursing courses. Until nursing students are sensitized toward this new technology, they are not going to make carrier in telenursing. Apprehension and fear toward telemedicine can only be removed through providing the knowledge about telemedicine. There should be basic telemedicine nursing lesson in their course curriculum. Telenursing is still a remote concept in the developing countries, where focus is mainly on telemedicine.

1.6 Lack of IT champions: teletechnicians

Telemedicine is a hybrid system, which involves the medical as well as ICT domain for complete understanding of the telemedicine solutions and its delivery. There is a serious lack of such technical persons, who can run day-to-day business of telemedicine. To run any telemedicine system properly, trained technical manpower is required. There is lack of technical champions in the field of telemedicine in India, especially in the field of health care and only voluntary champions here and there are visible.

It is common fact that many provider physicians and clients cannot fix the technical problems arising from computer system and ICT network. So, for a proper and smooth functioning of telemedicine system, we need trained and expert manpower to establish a stable and continuous communication during teleconsultation [25]. Unfortunately, there is serious lack of such trained persons in the system in most of the developing countries.

There are very few institutions in developing countries, which train and develop this special group of technicians. It is very difficult to find a person who has undergone training in Medicine and in Information Technology.

1.6.1 Technological barriers

Technology itself is becoming a barrier in the development of telemedicine in developing countries. High cost of replacing the older technology is not affordable for many stakeholders.

1.7 Rapid upgradation of ICT

Due to rapid advancement of telemedicine technology, many state-of-the-art facilities and equipment (software and hardware) become obsolete and outdated.

A complex and often unwieldy technical infrastructure may yield disappointing evaluations until it becomes more ubiquitous and user-friendly [23]. People working with these outdated technologies become demotivated and frustrated and lose interest in providing services through old technology system. Government also finds it difficult to replace, which is easily due to lots of budgetary requirement for newer technology.

Failure of telemedicine network in Madhya Pradesh, India, is an important example, where Indian Space Research Organization (ISRO) sponsored equipment like camera, television sets and other equipment and software were not utilized for a longtime and became outdated and nonfunctional. Repair and replacement of these equipment and software are so costly that government is not willing to get it repaired and whole telemedicine network has collapsed [14].

Time gap between acquiring hardware and development of customized software is so large that by the time software is ready, the hardware becomes obsolete. This mismatch between software and hardware also create a bottleneck in the development of effective telemedicine solution.

1.8 Inadequate ICT infrastructure

Many developing countries have inadequate availability of Information and Communication Technology (ICT) such as computers, Internet network, printers, and electricity for proper implementation and running of telemedicine program. Internet access and power supply are other issues related to failure of telemedicine network in rural and remote locations [14, 18, 24]. One of the important hurdles to effective delivery of telemedicine solution to rural and remote locations in developing countries is incomplete and insufficient ICT infrastructure.

1.9 Initial huge start-up cost of ICT infrastructure

Telemedicine set up can deploy varieties of information and communication technologies (ICTs) for transmitting information through texts, pictures, audios, and videos to a variety of healthcare providers. Cost depends on the type of ICT being used for the start-up. For setting an audio visual ICT platform for teleconsultation needs huge investment. Budgetary constraints become a major barrier in the development of telemedicine network in developing countries [7, 18, 19, 24]. A sustainable financial support is needed to purchase, deploy, operate, and maintain the sophisticated telemedicine platform [19]. Telecommunication expenses, training of service providers and clients, and need for newer ICT platforms require most of the expenditure.

1.10 Low Internet connectivity

Most of the telemedicine applications require a high speed and reliable Internet bandwidth to run smoothly. Tele-surgery, real time tele-ophthalmology, real time tele-radiology, and emergency consultation are some examples of such applications [25]. Unreliable and low wideband Internet pose barriers in smooth delivery of telemedicine service.

For real-time teleconsultations between providers and clients, there is a need for reliable and high speed Internet availability. Internet coverage is still bottleneck in many developing countries, especially in rural and remote areas. Most rural areas do not have the financial capital to independently invest in a broadband network that would provide high-speed Internet to their inhabitants. Telecommunications ("telecom") companies are the primary providers of high-speed Internet, but they invest very little in rural areas because such investments are not as profitable [26].

Internet connectivity for transmitting patients' files, records, pictures, and videos are still limited in many areas, including in China, India, Indonesia, the Philippines, and Vietnam [27]. Recently, it has been observed that Internet access is growing and also the cost of Internet is coming down, which is a good sign for the development of telemedicine on developing countries.

1.10.1 Legal barriers

Telemedicine practices has eliminated many physical and emotional barriers to healthcare seeking but have raised many legal and ethical issues, which are normally not encountered during traditional healthcare delivery. Legal considerations are a major obstacle to telemedicine uptake [8, 21, 28].

1.11 Online prescription

There is no legal framework of e-prescription, digital prescription, or mobile-based SMS prescription. Digital prescriptions are not approved and accepted by Medical Council of India (MCI) or any other regulatory authority [8]. Online prescribing policies vary across the countries and across the states within countries.

Concerns have been raised over various issues like whether an appropriate patient-provider relationship has been established, lack of an adequate physical examination of the patient, accuracy of the patient's history given the self-reporting of the patient over a telehealth connection, and not meeting state medical board licensing requirements [29]. There is no standardized legal framework to protect practitioners as well as clients for online prescriptions in developing countries.

1.12 Malpractice liability

Most of the doctors are afraid of Consumer Protection Act due to malpractice-related issues. There is a lack of specific standard operating procedures (SOPs)/ guidelines for the telemedicine practice [8]. Legal issues surrounding patient privacy, safety, security, and confidentiality also play vital role in teleconsultation. Very little information exists on the extent of malpractice liability and telehealth [29]. Medical malpractice-related legal issues should be identified and addressed for smooth practice of telemedicine.

1.13 Licensing of telemedicine/telehealth service providers

Highly sophisticated, safe, secure, and speedy teleconsultations have reduced the distance barrier in healthcare seeking and have improved the healthcare access. In order to avoid malpractice in telemedicine, healthcare professionals should be specifically trained for telemedicine as they do for traditional medicine [30]. Poor availability of experts and trained professions raises legal implications and warrants licensing of telemedicine providers.

The responsibility of licensing to telemedicine providers falls under the purview of the state licensing councils or boards of a particular country. These policies governing telemedicine and physician licensure vary widely across the country [29].

Licensing ensures that physicians meet academic and clinical competence standards for the telemedicine practice. It protects public from unqualified and substandard physicians and healthcare professorial. Licensing also helps to enforce continuing standards [31].

1.14 Informed consent before teleconsultation

Need for a prior written or verbal informed consent for any telemedicine consultation and treatment misrepresents telemedicine as a different form of service, rather than as a useful tool that enhances diagnostic and treatment services.

Healthcare providers need to have a clear understanding of what their legal and ethical responsibilities are. Similarly, patients must receive the protection of adequate standards of care and know that the person to whom they are entrusting their health has the proper qualifications [31].

The lack of clear-cut legal guidelines, rules, and regulations hinders the telemedicine to improve healthcare access and healthcare quality through information and communication technology [31].

1.14.1 Financial barriers to telemedicine development

Although telemedicine can be leveraged to increase access to care and reduce the cost of care but that is mainly true for the user's point of view. Story is different if we look from the side of providers or healthcare organizations. For establishing a telemedicine unit, it needs lots of financial investment. It becomes more difficult for the developing countries to allocate huge budget for the investment in telemedicine.

Establishing and operating a "Telemedicine Unit" require purchasing the equipment needed to setup the system at both provider's and consumer's end (in the hospital, clinic, or pharmacy); maintaining the equipment; training the physicians and local healthcare workers on the technology; and compensating the physicians. There are many other costs are involve in delivering teleconsultation like payment of Internet and electricity bills, salary of support staff, other recurring costs etc.

These total costs are so high that many proposals of establishing or starting telemedicine program never take off, or even if it starts, it dies soon and cannot sustain on a long-term basis. Many telemedicine pilot projects have failed because of high maintenance cost [14].

The costs of telemedicine are often high in developing countries, because of low awareness between both patients and local healthcare workers, low information technology literacy, and limited access to infrastructure and technology [27]. Telemedicine service providers are generally unable to bear all costs alone and expect government or development partner to support financially for the sustainability of the telemedicine projects.

Most of the telemedicine solutions and programs tend to be government funded, at least in their initial phases. Due to some reasons, if government stops funding, the system becomes unsustainable as there is no alternative business model. So dependency on public support is another financial barrier in the development of telemedicine in developing countries [27].

Cost incurred in purchase, installation, and maintenance of telemedicine services (telemedicine and communication equipment) are very high and do not give proper return on investment (ROI), so there is less economic benefits to the practitioners, which leads to the bankruptcy and closure of many health facilities in rural communities and also prevents further telemedicine expansion to communities needing specialized services [32]. Insurance companies do not reimburse the teleconsultation bills and payments, which further force the practitioners to stop the telemedicine services. Many hospitals and clinics perceive that telemedicine solutions are too expensive to implement.

1.15 Reimbursement and insurance barriers

Reimbursement of telemedicine services has been reported as one of the important barriers in developed countries [17, 22, 33, 34]. When patient avails healthcare services through telemedicine system, insurance claim may not cover the cost of care as it is not delivered through traditional healthcare system. Such discrimination seldom occurs in developing countries, where health insurance is still a rare commodity [30].

1.15.1 Social barriers in the development of telemedicine

Social and culture milieu of the community and society of a particular country also creates lots of barriers in adapting, utilizing, and sustaining telemedicine services. The lack of ICT literacy, awareness, language barriers, and cultural gaps between the service providers and patients etc. are also major factors, which prevent further development and expansion of telemedicine network in developing countries.

1.16 Resistance to change

A lack of support to newer ICT tools has been observed from both parties (providers and users). Several studies have revealed that the resistance to change has been reported toward telemedicine from providers (physicians) as well as from users (clients/patients) for newer technology [14, 19, 25, 33, 35].

1.17 ICT literacy

In developing countries where general literacy is not even adequate, we can imagine the awareness level of population toward ITC literacy. Poor awareness toward modern technologies and their use in delivering health care seems to be a big barrier in developing countries. People in developing countries are not much aware about the benefits offered by telemedicine. Even physicians are short of IT knowledge and not updated. Poor awareness level creates fears and resistance toward ICT technology and create hurdle in the adoption and development of telemedicine. Age also plays an important role. Many older physicians do not feel comfortable dealing with ICT technology. Some patients, particularly older patients, are hesitant about the new technology.

Many healthcare professionals are not comfortable working with computers and modern gadgets and consider technology extra work for them. They also fear that telemedicine may lead to job loss or a reduction in their bedside presence [27, 33].

1.18 Lack of confidence

There is lack of confidence in patients about the outcome of telemedicine. It is difficult for them to believe that machine can provide healthcare demands without visiting physician face to face [25]. This cultural perception and attitude toward newer technology also possess threat to the development of telemedicine. Even many physicians also think that patient consultation and treatment are incomplete without touching the patient and prefer face-to-face consultation than remote consultation through ICT platform. Some medical practitioners do not want to opt telemedicine practice due to the fear of medical indemnity.

Barriers to adoption and sustainability of rural telehealth embody several factors that must be considered when planning, developing, implementing, and evaluating a rural telehealth program [32].

1.19 Industry-oriented telemedicine

There are three players in the telemedicine viz. physicians as service providers, IT Industry as supplier of technology, and public as user. One of the major hurdles of development of telemedicine in developing countries is the passiveness of provider physician and users.

Most of the telemedicine tools and technologies are developed and supplied by the developed countries and they have strong market influence in the developing countries. IT industry people are very active and try to influence policy makers and administrators in the health system to sell their IT technology (telemedicine-related hardware and software). Their focus is only to sell and install the telemedicine tools and equipment and leave the system for the physician to run.

Failure is bound to happen if providers and users are not taken into account while developing the telemedicine platform. For example, in Madhya Pradesh, India, ISRO and top-level administrators at ministry level decided to implement telemedicine solutions across the state but it failed badly as there were no takers at ground level. Physicians were not convinced and adequately trained for newer technology and public as a user was not aware about the benefit of the platform [14].

2. Conclusion

Health care in developing countries is in the midst of a paradigm shift, from a traditional provider-centered, disease-oriented approach to a patient-centered, health-management model. Telemedicine has influenced almost all aspects of healthcare and many success stories have reported the role of telemedicine in improving healthcare access, reducing cost of care, and enhancing the quality of care. Telemedicine could be an important tool in achieving healthcare coordination and reducing healthcare disparities.

Despite of so much development and successful work in the field of telemedicine, it has yet to become integral part of healthcare system. Success of telemedicine only depends when it becomes integral part of healthcare delivery system and not as a stand-alone project. Now, it is time to take telemedicine from pilot mode to routine operational mode in mainstream health services delivery system.

There is tremendous pressure on governments to provide accessible affordable and quality healthcare to its people. Only alternative and innovative methods like telemedicine can help to fulfill this gap. Current status of telemedicine in developing countries is not very satisfactory and passing through a stage of crisis. This chapter has explored the various barriers in the development of telemedicine in developing countries.

These various barriers mentioned above are impeding the speed of expansion of telemedicine in developing countries. It is now time to minimize the abovementioned barriers and remove the bottlenecks for smooth development of telemedicine network across the globe for the betterment of humanity.

Acknowledgements

The author would like to thank the Department of Public Health and Family Welfare Madhya Pradesh and National Health Mission Madhya Pradesh for providing funding support to conduct telemedicine evaluation survey from where experience has been shared here.

Conflict of interest

The author declares that he has no competing interest with anyone in publishing this chapter.

Notes/thanks/other declarations

No other declarations.

Author details

Surya Bali[1,2]*

1 Department of Community and Family Medicine, All India Institute of Medical Sciences Bhopal, Bhopal, Madhya Pradesh, India

2 Telemedicine Centre, All India Institute of Medical Sciences Bhopal, Bhopal, Madhya Pradesh, India

*Address all correspondence to: surya.cfm@aiimsbhopal.edu.in

References

[1] Kurji Z, Premani ZS, Mithani Y. Review and analysis of quality healthcare system enhancement in developing countries. The Journal of the Pakistan Medical Association. 2015;**65**(7):6

[2] Peters. Poverty and Access to Health Care in Developing Countries. Annals of the New York Academy of Sciences [Internet]. 2008. Wiley Online Library. Available from: https://nyaspubs.onlinelibrary.wiley.com/doi/epdf/10.1196/annals.1425.011 [Cited: September 16, 2018]

[3] Reerink IH, Sauerborn R. Quality of primary health care in developing countries: Recent experiences and future directions. International Journal for Quality in Health Care. 1996;**8**(2):131-139

[4] Haddad S, Fournier P. Quality, cost and utilization of health services in developing countries. A longitudinal study in Zaïre. Social Science & Medicine. 1995;**40**(6):743-753

[5] Puteh SEW, Almualm Y. Catastrophic Health Expenditure Among Developing Countries. Health Systems and Policy Research [Internet]. 2017;4(1). Available from: http://www.hsprj.com/abstract/catastrophic-health-expenditure-among-developing-countries-18514.html [Cited: September 16, 2018]

[6] Jacobs B, Ir P, Bigdeli M, Annear PL, Van Damme W. Addressing access barriers to health services: An analytical framework for selecting appropriate interventions in low-income Asian countries. Health Policy and Planning. 2012;**27**(4):288-300

[7] Chiang C, Adly Labeeb S, Higushi M, Ghardes Mohamed A, Aoyama A. Barriers to the use of basic health services among women in rural southern Egypt (upper Egypt). Nagoya Journal of Medical Science. 2013;**75**(3-4):225-231

[8] Bali S. Enhancing the reach of health care through telemedicine: Status and new possibilities in developing countries. In Health Care Delivery and Clinical Science: Concepts, Methodologies, Tools, and Applications, ed. Information Resources Management Association. Accessed December 03, 2018:1382-1397. DOI: 10.4018/978-1-5225-3926-1.ch069

[9] Telemedicine, Telehealth, and Health Information Technology an ATA Issue Paper Patient Care Health Provider [Internet]. Available from: http://www.who.int/goe/policies/countries/usa_support_tele.pdf [Cited: September 16, 2018]

[10] WHO. Telehealth [Internet]. WHO. Available from: http://www.who.int/sustainable-development/health-sector/strategies/telehealth/en/ [Cited: September 16, 2018]

[11] World Health Organization, editor. Telemedicine: Opportunities and developments in member states: Report on the second Global survey on eHealth [Internet]. 2010. Geneva, Switzerland: World Health Organization. 93 p. (Global Observatory for eHealth Series). Available from: http://www.who.int/goe/publications/goe_telemedicine_2010.pdf

[12] Alghamdi M, Gashgari H, Househ M. A systematic review of mobile health technology use in developing countries. Studies in Health Technology and Informatics. 2015;**213**:223-226

[13] Bali S, Singh AJ. Mobile phone consultation for community health care in rural north India. Journal

of Telemedicine and Telecare. 2007;**13**(8):421-424

[14] Bali S, Gupta A, Khan A, Pakhare A. Evaluation of telemedicine centres in Madhya Pradesh, Central India. Journal of Telemedicine and Telecare. 2016;**22**(3):183-188

[15] Bagayoko CO, Müller H, Geissbuhler A. Assessment of internet-based tele-medicine in Africa (the RAFT project). Computerized Medical Imaging and Graphics. 2006;**30**(6):407-416

[16] Doarn CR. The last challenges and barriers to the development of telemedicine programs. Studies in Health Technology and Informatics. 2008;**131**:45-54

[17] Moffatt JJ, Eley DS. Barriers to the up-take of telemedicine in Australia–A view from providers. Rural and Remote Health. 2011;**11**(2):1581

[18] Sorwar G, Rahamn MM, Uddin R, Hoque MR. Cost and time effectiveness analysis of a telemedicine service in Bangladesh. Studies in Health Technology and Informatics. 2016;**231**:127-134

[19] Alaboudi A, Atkins A, Sharp B, Balkhair A, Alzahrani M, Sunbul T. Barriers and challenges in adopting Saudi telemedicine network: The perceptions of decision makers of healthcare facilities in Saudi Arabia. Journal of Infection and Public Health. 2016;**9**(6): 725-733

[20] Zanaboni P, Lettieri E. Institutionalizing telemedicine applications: The challenge of legitimizing decision-making. Journal of Medical Internet Research. 2011;**13**(3):e72. https://www.jmir.org/2011/3/e72. DOI: 10.2196/jmir.1669 PMID: 21955510. PMCID: PMC322217

[21] Alghatani KM. Telemedicine Implementation: Barriers and Recommendations. Journal of Scientific Research and Studies.2016;**3**(7):140-145

[22] JahangirAlam M. E-governance in Bangladesh: Present problems and possible suggestions for future development. International Journal of Applied Information Systems. 2012;**4**(8):21-25

[23] Field MJ. Telemedicine: A Guide to Assessing Telecommunications for Health Care [Internet]. Institute of Medicine. Available from: https://www.nap.edu/read/5296/chapter/7 [Cited: September 16, 2018]

[24] Hoque MR, Mazmum MFA, Bao Y. e-Health in Bangladesh: Current status, challenges, and future direction. International Technology Management Review. 2014;**4**(2):87-96

[25] Hassibian MR, Hassibian S. Telemedicine acceptance and implementation in developing countries: Benefits, categories, and barriers. Razavi International Journal of Medicine. 2016;**4**(3):1-7

[26] Perkins A. A Cure to Rural Healthcare Access: Telemedicine, High-Speed Internet, and Local Government [Internet]. Harvard Journal of Law and Technology. Available from: https://jolt.law.harvard.edu/digest/a-cure-to-rural-healthcare-access-telemedicine-high-speed-internet-and-local-government [Cited: September 16, 2018]

[27] Endeva, Insight A, Hazarika M.Using Telemedicine to Treat Patients in Underserved Areas: Health Telemedicine Case [Internet]. 2017. World Bank Group. Available from: https://www.innovationpolicyplatform.org/system/files/2_%20Health%20

Telemedicine%20Case_Jun15.pdf [Cited: September 18, 2018]

[28] Stanberry B. Telemedicine: Barriers and opportunities in the 21st century. Journal of Internal Medicine. 2000;**247**(6):615-628

[29] Common Legal Barriers. Center for Connected Health Policy [Internet]. Available from: http://www.cchpca.org/common-legal-barriers [Cited: September 17, 2018]

[30] Combi C, Pozzani G, Pozzi G. Telemedicine for developing countries. Applied Clinical Informatics. 2016;7(4):1025-1050

[31] Daley HA. Telemedicine: The invisible legal barriers to the health care of the future. Annals of Health Law. 2000;**9**:35

[32] Alverson DC, Shannon S, Sullivan E, Prill A, Effertz G, Helitzer D, et al. Telehealth in the trenches: Reporting back from the frontlines in rural America. Telemedicine Journal and e-Health. 2004;**10**(Suppl 2):S-95-S109

[33] Bishop TF, Press MJ, Mendelsohn JL, Casalino LP. Electronic communication improves access, but barriers to its widespread adoption remain. Health Affairs | Project HOPE. 2013;**32**(8):1361-1367

[34] Wootton R, Vladzymyrskyy A, Zolfo M, Bonnardot L. Experience with Low-cost Telemedicine in Three Different Settings. Recommendations Based on a Proposed Framework for Network Performance Evaluation. Glob Health Action [Internet]. 2011;4. Available from: https://www.ncbi.nlm.nih.gov/pmc/articles/PMC3234078/ [Cited: September 16, 2018]

[35] Ghani MKA, Jaber MM, Herman NS. Barriers faces telemedicine implementation in the developing countries: Toward building iraqi telemedicine framework. ARPN Journal of Engineering and Applied Sciences. 2015;**10**(4):6

Chapter 4

The Advent of Application Specific Integrated Circuits (ASIC)-MEMS within the Medical System

Jian-Chiun Liou

Abstract

Medical healthcare has become one of the fastest growing and largest industries in the world. More and more people are aware of the precious and important life. At the same time, personal disposable income increases and awareness of disease prevention increases. It allows the healthcare industry to maintain high growth rates. Micro-electro- mechanical systems (MEMS) is one of the most revolutionary semiconductor components. The advent of Application Specific Integrated Circuits (ASIC)-MEMS has created a new era for the healthcare industry. The medical Micro LED detects the blood vessel position with the emission light source and repositions the blood flow state of the blood vessel. Micro LED mainly uses the MEMS micro-fabrication technology to micronize, array, and thin film the traditional LED crystal film. This article will explore how to use MEMS wafers to redefine the needs of the healthcare market and open up new growth opportunities for healthcare applications. With the shift from first-hand medical devices from the hospital business to personal use, miniaturization, economics, reliability and battery life have become new demands in the healthcare market.

Keywords: ASIC, MEMS, medical system

1. Introduction

Biometric technology has freed people from cumbersome passwords and cluttered IC cards. Among them, the finger vein identification technology is also referred to by the industry as the world's top biometric identification technology. Its misrecognition rate was only 0.0001%, far below the 0.001% of the fingerprint and 1.3% of the face. Although fingerprint recognition technology and face recognition are developing rapidly, there are some flaws [1–12].

In addition to the identification technology itself needs to be improved, some problems that are difficult to avoid, such as being affected by human body temperature. Some unexpected situations such as peeling, injury, etc. will affect the ability to identify. In this case, finger vein recognition technology came into being. It is referred to by the industry as the world's top biometric technology. It is understood that fingerprint, face, iris and other identity recognition systems are good. However, there are still some technical loopholes. As long as it fingerprints its own fingerprints, it allows others to punch cards. Furthermore, if a fugitive turns his face through plastic surgery, then the security measures for customs, airports, and other public places will be like dummy. In addition, iris recognition technology is extremely accurate. However, it is powerless for patients with blind or eye diseases. In addition, iris recognition technology requires expensive cameras for image acquisition, which is costly and difficult to use in a wide range of applications. In Asia, iris recognition technology is difficult to promote. Another important factor is that the technology is very difficult to identify with dark eyes. The sound will have a big contrast with usual. At this point, the voice recognition system is likely to be misjudged or unrecognizable. As a "live recognition" technology, finger vein recognition is via a finger vein identifier. It obtains individual finger vein maps, stores characteristic values, and then matches them for personal identification. The basic principle is to use the red blood cells in veins to absorb this characteristic of specific near-infrared rays. The finger is irradiated with near-infrared light, and the light transmitted by the finger is sensed by an image sensor. It acquires the vein image inside the finger to perform biometric identification. The key is the hemoglobin in the erythrocytes flowing through the veins. It absorbs near-infrared rays near the wavelength of 700–1000 nm. It causes less transmission of near-infrared rays in the vein portion. When near-infrared light is transmitted, the veins are highlighted on the image sensed by the image sensor. The muscles, bones, and other parts of the fingers are weakened. This gives clear images of veins. Finger vein recognition technology uses the texture of the finger veins for authentication. It is harmless to the human body, and it is not easily stolen or forged [13–19].

In 1993, scholars Allen and Murray used an Artificial Neural Network (ANN) algorithm to classify PPG waveform shapes (SI) in patients with foot lesions. The results showed a 90% accuracy and the degree of vascular lesions in the lower extremities could be identified [20–25]. In 2008, scholars Allen et al. combined the correlation between ECG waveforms and the PPG waveforms of the temporal limbs of the lower extremities, and proposed quantification of the number of parameters used as the basis for the degree of vascular lesions [26–28].

The human body itself is a chemical sensor and has a variety of chemical sensing functions. It includes taste, smell, hormonal receptors of the endocrine system, neurochemical transmission materials of the nerve conduction system, and the like.

Chemosensory devices are bio-technical methods for obtaining bioactive molecules in the human body. It enables chemical reactions with molecular recognition materials of specific substances. It converts this reaction into an electronic signal via a converter and outputs graphic information to medical personnel for interpretation. For example, respiratory testing, immunological testing, genetic screening, drug tracking, etc. are all commonly used chemical sensing methods. Its main sensing biochemical parameters include: respiratory gas composition, blood, blood glucose, pH, and chromatography. BioMEMS covers biotechnology, nanomaterials, and MEMS integration technologies. In addition to the general miniaturization of biomedical testing instruments, it also contributes to the development of smaller, lower power implantable biomedical sensors. It allows patients with chronic conditions that require long-term physiological monitoring to be used more comfortably and conveniently.

Moreover, it utilizes a microelectromechanical process compatible with complementary metal oxide semiconductors (CMOS). BioMEMS integrates sophisticated application IC circuits and RF chips. It not only improves product functionality, but also transmits and analyzes biomedical test data. It is conducive to the establishment of a complete medical information network, or even to achieve remote care services [29–31]. In this study, the medical Micro LED scans the blood vessel position with the emission light source and repositions the blood flow state of the blood vessel. This study included system design, Micro LED arrays combined with CMOS processes, and post-assembly assembly measurements.

2. Architecture

BioMEMS biomedical sensors are mainly using microelectronics technology to miniaturize large-scale detection instruments. The sensor's architecture combines microelectronics, microfluidics, and biodetection technologies. It is used with physical or chemical converters to convert biochemical parameters into electronic signals. Finally, digital output is used to present relevant detection information in graphic form. It is provided to users (biochemical researchers, medical professionals, patients or their families, etc.) for interpretation. The physical sensor is mainly a measure of the physical characteristics of the body itself. The sensing parameters include: size or shape change, force/force distance value, speed/acceleration, temperature, pressure, and flow. It applies these physical parameters to design a BioMEMS sensor that can sense changes in subtle physical quantities. It measures body reactions such as muscle contraction, blood pressure, body temperature, blood flow rate, electrocardiogram, and vision.

The medical Micro LED scans the blood vessel position with the emission light source and repositions the blood flow state of the blood vessel. Micro LED mainly uses the MEMS micro-fabrication technology to micronize, array, and thin film the traditional LED crystal film. It uses a large amount of transfer technology to mass transfer the crystalline film to the circuit board. It uses physical deposition to make the protective layer and finally completes the package. Among them, the key core technologies mainly include two steps: the micro-processing technology and the massive transfer technology.

Inductively Coupled Plasma Ion Etching (ICP) was used on the epitaxial thin film layer of the LED. It directly forms a micron-sized Micro LED epitaxial thin film structure. The fixed pitch of this structure is the required pitch for displaying the pixels. It bonds the LED wafer (including the epitaxial layer and the substrate) directly to the driver circuit substrate, and finally peels the substrate using a physical or chemical mechanism. It only has 4–5 μm Micro LED epitaxial thin film structure on the drive circuit substrate to form display pixels.

a. Define a pattern of metal bumps using photo resists in the open area of the exposed SiNx dielectric protection layer. It produces fine pitch In bumps with thermal evaporation squares. Subsequently, the FC-150 die bonder was used to thermo-bond the LED die onto the CMOS substrate, followed by an under-fill to fix the micro-die array.

b. The native GaAs substrate of the red LED is removed by wet etching. It uses an ammonia aqueous solution ($NH_4OH:H_2O_2$ = 1:10) soaked at 50° for 30 minutes to remove the GaAs substrate. All active 192 × 64 LED microchip array device manufacturing processes have been completed. The structure of the micro-chip LED array device is shown in **Figure 1**.

The purpose of pulling the common N metal electrode with a redistribution layer to the same height as the area of the Micro LED Pixel is to improve the contact yield of the In bump bonding-induced CMOS substrate. In biomedical applications, optical/optical chemical sensors using optical principles are common methods in the field of biology. It uses the biomedical detection method of the optical principle. It mainly utilizes the self-luminous effect of the biomolecule itself or the extra light

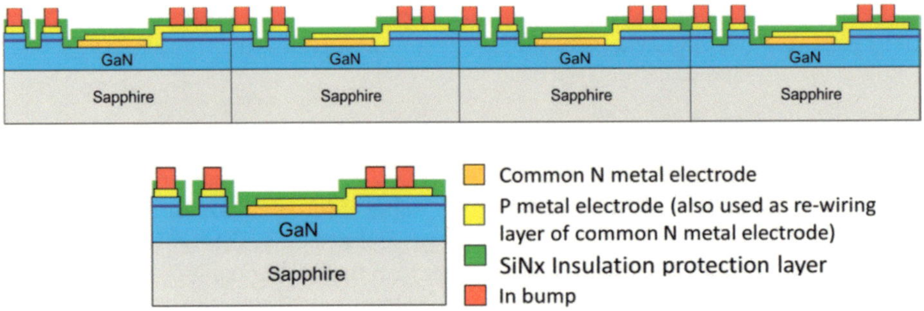

Figure 1.
Blue and green light resolution 192 × 64, pixel cycle 19.2 μm linear arrangement of micro-crystals LED array element schematic diagram.

effect induced by the extraneous molecule, so that the optical signal is obtained and the quantitative optical measurement method is used. It tests the various optical signals that have been obtained. This method is also conducive to detection under an optical microscope. Spectral analysis is a common detection method for optical/optical chemical sensors. Spectral analysis is a non-destructive, real-time detection technique with a wide spectral range. It is not disturbed by electrical noise. Therefore, multiple parameters can be detected at the same time. It has the advantages of being quick, simple and accurate. BioMEMS Cooperates with ICT technology; it uses BioMEMS sensors made by MEMS technology. In addition to its small size, it is easy to integrate with integrated circuits. It has the advantages of high integration in related biomedical detection digital signal processors (DSPs), analog/digital conversion chips and other circuits. Therefore, in data acquisition and calculation, it can have a higher resolution than previous detection instruments and can process multiple data at the same time. CMOS improves integration, microcomputer-based sensors for biomedical applications have been introduced into the CMOS standard process to help integrate biosensing devices with related measurement circuits. It can further integrate heterogeneous circuits such as RF chip, biomedical detection DSP, and analog/digital conversion chip in System in Package (SiP) mode. Sensors can include multi-applications such as specimen import/export, specimen sensing, signal interpretation, data storage, wireless transmission, and instant exception alerts. In addition, BioMEMS biomedical sensors can be manufactured in large quantities through CMOS standardization processes. Significantly reduce production costs, in addition to help in some detection applications. It can produce disposable products to reduce the risk of cross-contamination of specimens. Increased efficiency/accuracy, in clinical applications, especially in dealing with various acute and chronic diseases, it measures the changes of various biomedical detection signals in the physiological system in real time. It is often the decision-making basis for diagnosis and treatment. BioMEMS sensors constructed using MEMS technology. With the development of digitalization, its sensors can quickly perform functions such as sensory sensing, data storage, and abnormal warning. In addition to providing more information for professional judgment, it can conduct continuous monitoring and data comparison. It helps the medical staff to detect abnormal reactions of the patient as soon as possible so that appropriate medical action can be taken immediately.

The miniaturization of BioMEMS allows the device to be worn or implanted in the body to enable continuous monitoring and comprehensive prevention. It immediately provides the patient's physiological condition to the medical staff, enabling the patient's condition to be diagnosed and treated promptly. Furthermore, medical staff can also help improve the lifestyle of the patient in view of the accumulated

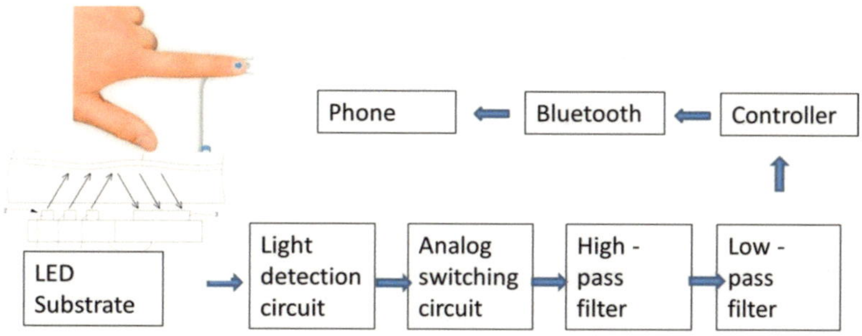

Figure 2.
The application specific integrated circuits (ASIC)-MEMS within the medical system.

information. The wireless transmission accelerates data updates and uses wireless technology to transmit detection data for various care devices such as thermometers, scales, sphygmomanometers, blood glucose detectors, and electrocardiograms. It is applied to medical examinations in general medical institutions. It can achieve real-time data consolidation and instant medical diagnostic operations. **Figure 2** is the application specific integrated circuits (ASIC)-MEMS within the medical system.

Infrared light has strong penetrating power on human skin and subcutaneous tissue. External effects of infrared radiation on the human body can increase the temperature of skin and subcutaneous tissue. It promotes blood circulation and metabolism and promotes human health.

Infrared physiotherapy has been confirmed clinically for the thermal effects, anti-inflammatory effects and regeneration of tissue. It is usually treated with direct irradiation of the lesion.

Near-infrared micro-irradiation therapy has a significant improvement in microcirculation. Especially in the micro-flow state improved significantly. The performance of the capillary blood flow after irradiation was accelerated, and the red blood cell aggregation was reduced. The phenomenon of hyperemia in the inferior venous plexus of the finger decreases or disappears. Therefore, it has a positive effect on improving the nutrition, metabolism, repair and function of body tissues and important organs. The mechanism by which infrared light produces secondary effects on the human body is not yet fully understood. The frequency of sound waves is higher than 20,000 Hz, which is called "ultrasonics". Ultrasonic mechanical vibration is used in medical treatment and is called "ultrasonic treatment". The medical behavior of implanting organisms with ultrasonic energy is "supersonic free penetration therapy." Ultrasound diagnosis uses ultrasound as a part of the biological scan to detect pathological changes. Ultrasonic waves can also be mixed with other different currents if needed. It not only can easily detect the sensing area of the tissue of the birth object, but also can be used for fixed-point treatment.

3. Fabrication

In this study, blue-green, red-colored and red-colored LED epitaxial wafers were used for the process development of micro-chip LED array elements. The process-related steps were as follows: the optimization process was developed, and the process steps were described briefly.

1. Blue and green GaN-based microchip LED array device manufacturing process:

a. Defining the P-type metal contact electrode area on the surface of the P-type semiconductor layer with a photoresist using a yellow lithography process. It uses an E-beam evaporator to deposit 225 nm thick indium tin oxide ITO as a P-type ohmic contact metal. The characteristic resistance value of about 1E-2 Ω-cm^2 can be obtained after 1 minute treatment at an annealing temperature of 600°C. P-type ohmic contact metal on the blue and green light surface of the wafer is formed with photoresist on it to define the microchip LED Mesa platform pattern. It uses RIE to etch the photoresist pattern and transfer it to the surface of the blue and green light-emitting wafers. After removing the excess photoresist layer, the active layer of the well is exposed to the N-type semiconductor layer to complete the Mesa platform definition. The etching depth is about 0.8 μm.

b. Define an N-type metal contact electrode pattern with photoresist on the N-type semiconductor layer exposed by the etching. It uses an E-beam evaporator to deposit approximately 500 nm of titanium/gold (Ti/Au = 2000 Å/3000 Å) as an N-type ohmic contact metal electrode with a characteristic resistance of 1E-4 Ω-cm^2.

c. SiNx dielectric protection layer grown 300° PECVD with a thickness of 0.3 μm to ensure the position of the indium ball when indium bumps are reflowed into indium balls. It uses a photoresist on the SiNx to define the dielectric protection layer opening pattern in a yellow lithography process. The pattern is etched to remove the SiNx material from the area to the P-type metal contact electrode exposed for subsequent metal bump fabrication.

d. Define a pattern of metal bumps with photo-resist exposed areas of the exposed SiNx dielectric protection layer. It produces fine pitch indium bumps in thermal vapor deposition squares. Subsequently, the LED die was thermocompression bonded to the CMOS substrate with an FC-150 die bonder. Subsequent fabrications are filled under-fills to hold the microcrystal arrays. It completes all 192 × 64 LED microchip array active device processes.

e. It is to increase the difficulty of subsequent metal bump manufacturing process. It utilizes Dow Chemical's BCB-4026 material. The planarization

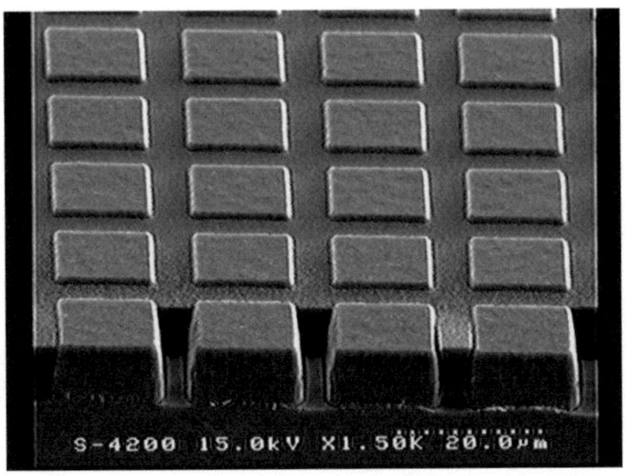

Figure 3.
SEM observation of the flattened coating of the green microcrystalline LED array with BCB.

coating is performed on the green light-emitting wafers that have been etched on the micro-chip LED array platform. It uses etching back to etch the BCB flat layer to the surface of the green light micro LED Mesa platform. It completes the planarization of the surface of the epitaxial wafer with the aforementioned insulating trenches, as shown in **Figure 3**.

4. Experiment and results

This is a micro-LED MEMS process combined with a CMOS substrate. The whole process requires the process of the clean room. Yellow light process developer causes a total N metal electrode surface damage. Therefore, when the common N metal electrode rewiring process is performed, the rewiring layer is stripped from the common N metal electrode. The ohmic metal contact electrode materials corresponding to the P-type and N-type semiconductor materials in the LED device manufacturing process are not the same. When the two metals are vapor-deposited, the heights of the bumps corresponding to the P-type and N-type regions are different when the indium bumps required for the subsequent fine-pitch bonding are produced due to different thicknesses of the metal plating films. This may affect the yield of LED die bonding with CMOS substrate metal. Therefore, the micro-chip LED array element prepared in this study extends the N-type ohmic contact electrode from the N-type semiconductor region to the LED platform in a metal rerouting (RDL) manner. This can improve the above problems. However, due to the different materials of P-type and N-type metals, the interface may be oxidized or etched and bombarded between two metal materials. As a result, the metal laminate is peeled off. Therefore, to improve this problem, the process steps are simplified in this process. The N-type metal extended LED platform is coated with a P-type ohmic contact electrode on the LED die array area. Afterwards, the N-type metal is directly self-interconnected. This avoids the problem of interface peeling between the two metal coatings.

The process result of the micro-chip LED array is shown in **Figure 4**. The difference between the blue and green light microchip LED array elements and the red light microchip LED array elements is only the depth of the platform etching and the BCB planarization coating process.

The I-V electrical test was performed on the blue and green microcrystalline LED arrays prepared as described above. The test results are as follows:

1. Blue-light micro-crystal LED array elements: VF ~ 2.9–3.1 V@20 mA/cm^2.

2. Green-light micro-crystal LED array element: VF ~ 3.1–3.4 V@20 mA/cm^2.

The Micro LED die is transferred to the circuit board in a large amount, and the brightness and contrast can be improved by integrating the micro lens array. An array of these display images, the Micro LED panel as shown in **Figure 5**, has scanning blood vessel positions and performs blood vessel product (PPG) detection.

At present, the reflective heart beat oxygen sensor can be divided into three types according to different light sources. The green LED mainly penetrates the skin to detect contraction and relaxation of the micro-vessels. It measures the heart rate through the vascular volume change calculation. The red and infrared LEDs are compared using different intensity of the two penetrating light sources. Because the absorption of light by oxygen and carbon dioxide in the blood is not the same, after optical signal processing, the value of hemorrhagic oxygen concentration can be converted as shown in **Figures 6** and **7**. In addition, blood pressure and blood concentration can also be measured by measuring blood oxygen content or skin conductivity.

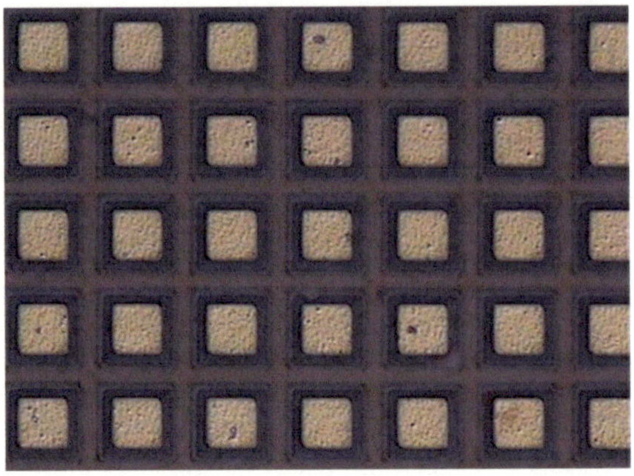

Figure 4.
Blue and green light resolution 192 × 64, pixel cycle 19.2 μm linear arrangement of micro-crystal LED array elements OM observation photo.

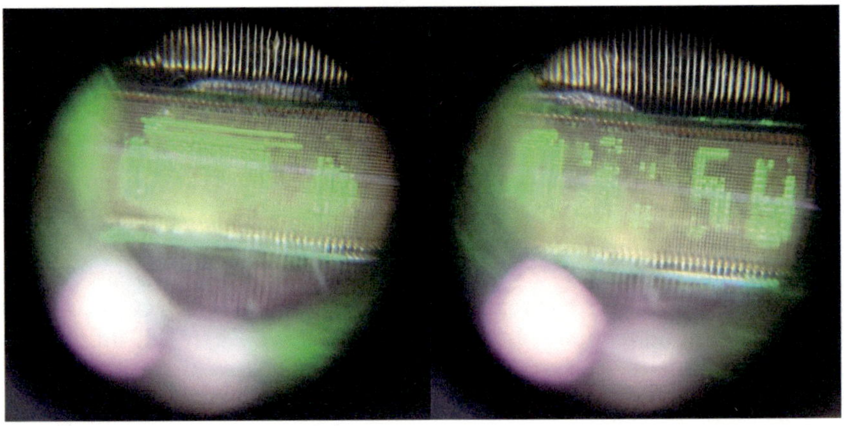

Figure 5.
Micro LED panel image photo.

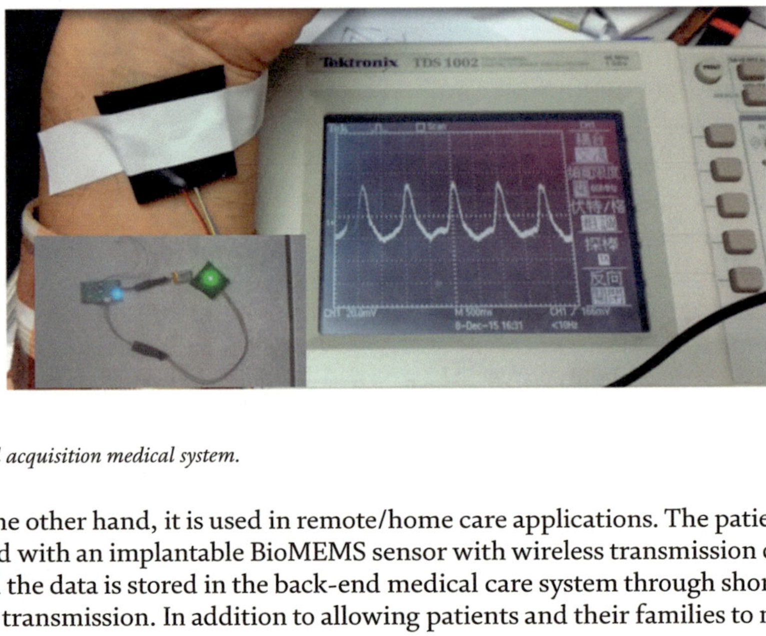

Figure 6.
PPG signal acquisition medical system.

On the other hand, it is used in remote/home care applications. The patient is equipped with an implantable BioMEMS sensor with wireless transmission capabilities, and the data is stored in the back-end medical care system through short-range wireless transmission. In addition to allowing patients and their families to manage

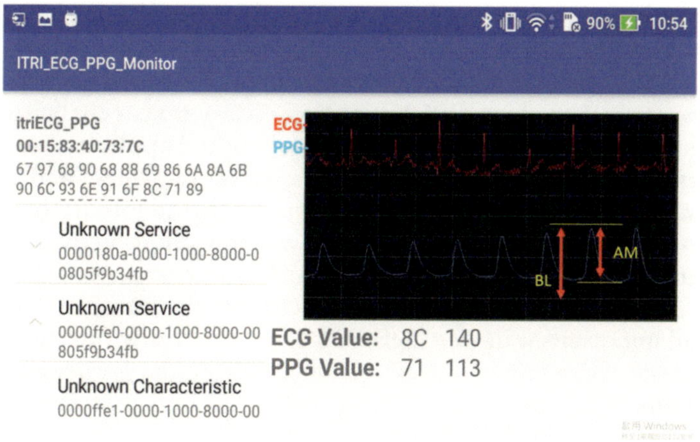

Figure 7.
ECG & PPG signal.

their own health, after a long time statistical analysis and analysis of their physiological testing data, the back-end medical system allows doctors to have more complete information for medical diagnosis. Some of the medical electronic components are planned to be integrated into personal terminal devices such as mobile phones, watches, clothing, and eyewear, to provide more complete and comprehensive care.

Aging society promotes medical electronics warming up, in the growing trend of social environmental development, such as population aging, cardiovascular disease and diabetes, self-monitoring and home care applications are gradually gaining popularity. Since the accuracy of the home-type biomedical detection instruments currently used in the market is not high, and it is inconvenient for patients to use and self-track management, the development of micro biomedical detection instruments using micro-electromechanical technology has become a goal of active development of relevant manufacturers.

The use of MEMS technology compatible with CMOS manufacturing to produce a new generation of BioMEMS biomedical sensors, in addition to being able to achieve miniaturization, due to the integration of related sensing elements, application of IC circuits, RF chips, etc. For technical and medical applications, improve its accuracy and the development of integrated applications. Looking ahead, the development of BioMEMS biomedical sensors not only facilitates the use of patients and healthcare personnel, but also integrates network transmission capabilities to further establish medical care networks and achieve the goal of remote/home care applications. Whether this goal can be achieved depends on whether the establishment of the industry's ecosystem and the evolution of technology are successful. ASIC-MEMS can be used by telemedicine providers in blood flow monitoring through Micro-LED arrays. Data can be uploaded to the cloud. Doctors in remote places can evaluate the data. The detection system provides feedback to local nurses and doctors. It is a way to increase the availability of the most advanced medical services in remote and rural areas using this technology. Detecting blood flow through ASIC-MEMS can reduce the cost of medicine. By doing so, it is possible to provide the world's most advanced medical services, including more developed countries and less developed countries.

5. Conclusions

In this article, we successfully designed and demonstrated an application specific integrated circuits (ASIC)-MEMS within the medical system. The Micro

LED die is transferred to the circuit board in a large amount, and the brightness and contrast can be improved by integrating the micro lens array. An array of these display images, the Micro LED panel, has scanning blood vessel positions and performs blood vessel product (PPG) detection. In low-power challenges remain, looking at the development of BioMEMS technology and applications, it can provide long-term monitoring applications that are more convenient and comfortable for patients with chronic diseases. However, there is still an important issue in the future development, is to achieve ultra-low power consumption. In order to reduce power consumption, relevant component manufacturers are actively developing low-power DSP and analog-digital converters (ADCs) dedicated to biomedical detection; and microsensor devices designed to automatically fine-tune the working cycle so that sensors can be used. ASIC-MEMS is best suited for use by telemedicine providers for blood flow monitoring through micro-LED arrays. This system is also the fastest to reach data can be uploaded to the cloud.

Acknowledgements

This work was supported by TMU106-AE1-B17.

Author biography

Dr. Jian-Chiun Liou received a Ph.D. degree from the Institute of Nanoengineering and Microsystems, National Tsing Hua University, Hsinchu, Taiwan, in 2009. He joined the Printing Technology Development and Manufacturing Section of the Optoelectronics and Systems Laboratories at the Industrial Technology Research Institute (ITRI), Hsinchu, in 1999, where he focused on the ink-jet printing system. Since 2005, he has been a Project Leader working on a new MEMS architecture design and display application in the Electronics and Optoelectronics Research Laboratories, ITRI. In August 2014, he joined the faculty of the National Kaohsiung University of Applied Sciences (KUAS). In August 2017, he has joined the School of Biomedical Engineering, Taipei Medical University (TMU), Taipei 11031, Taiwan. Currently, he is a Professor of School of Biomedical Engineering at the TMU. His research interests are in the fields of Optoelectronics, ASIC design, bio-chip technology, optical MEMS technology, integration of ink-jet printhead processes, and display technology. He is a holder of 71 patents on ink-jet printheads, MOEMS, MEMS, and has written more than 28 SCI Journal papers and 38 conference technical papers on MEMS, optical-N/MEMS, and display-related and micro-/nanofluidics related fields. He has also co-chaired many conference technical sessions and has been an invited speaker in many related events. In addition, he has performed the following tasks: Advance project leader (ITRI), SCI Journal paper reviewer (PIER, JEMWA, MEE), and Research fellow (NTHU). To add, Dr. Liou was the recipient of the following honors: ITRI/OES Research Achievement Award (2004), ITRI Research Paper Publication Award (2004), ITRI/EOL Research Achievement Award (Individual person Award, 2005), ITRI/EOL Outstanding Advanced Research Silver Award (2005), ITRI/EOL Research Achievement Award (2006), ITRI/EOL Patents Reviewer (2007), Outstanding Research Award (2007), ITRI/EOL Patents Reviewer (2008), Outstanding Research Award (2010), ITRI/EOL Patents Reviewer (2009), ITRI/EOL Outstanding Research Award (2010), International R&D 100 Awards (2010), 1st International Contest of Applications in Nano-Micro Technology Award (2010)—OPTO- MEMS Device Application, ITRI Paper Awards (2012), ITRI/EOL

Outstanding Advanced Research Silver Award (2013), International Inventor Prize (2014), Nation Academic Award (2014). 2014 Invention Lifetime Achievement Award. 2015 "Design and fabrication of Monolithic CMOS / MEMS system with HV-ESD Clamp protected inkjet printhead." 2015 International Contest Application Contest in Nano-Micro Technology (Alaska, USA) "iCAN'15 7th Special Prize" 2015 International Contest of Application in Nano-Micro Technology (iCAN'15). Who's Who in the World® 2016 (33rd Edition). In 2016, "The 16th Wang Golden silicon semiconductor design and application contest winners": An ASIC designed to spray liquid medical wisdom DNA gene sequencing system. 2016 Third Prize Award and Best Supervisors: Jian-Chiun Liou, 2016 iCAN'16 France 2016 International Contest of Application in Nano-Micro Technology (iCAN'16 ESIEE Paris, July 7th, 2016): The Glove. 2017 "iCAN'17 Third Prize Award, and Education Star Award 2017 International Contest of Application in Nano-Micro Technology (iCAN'17 BEIJING): Cloud Health Care (CHC). 2017 Teaching Excellence Teacher Award. August 2017 Transferred to Taipei Medical University for medical electronics related fields in-depth study. He is a member of the IEEE and a reviewer for more than 20 international journals including the Applied Physics Letters, JMEMS, Microfluidics and nano-fluidics, and micro-devices. He has also been a consultant to three Taiwanese companies.

Author details

Jian-Chiun Liou
School of Biomedical Engineering, Taipei Medical University, Taipei, Taiwan

*Address all correspondence to: jcliou@tmu.edu.tw

References

[1] Venkataramanan S, Kamble D, Bairolu A, Singh A, Rao R. A novel heart rate and non-invasive glucose measuring device. In: 2017 International Conference on Communication and Signal Processing (ICCSP), IEEE (Institute of Electrical and Electronics Engineers, Inc.). 2017. pp. 1796-1800

[2] Jayaprabha T, Suresh A. Blood flow, vein and nerves detector using an NIR sensor with RLS estimation for embedded signal processing. In: 2016 International Conference on Advanced Communication Control and Computing Technologies (ICACCCT), IEEE (Institute of Electrical and Electronics Engineers, Inc.). 2016. pp. 117-121

[3] Fragoon A, Mamoun A, Frah l, Alwahab SA. Biosynthesis of gold nanoparticle by fenugreek seed (trigonella foenum) extract. In: 2015 International Conference on Computing, Control, Networking, Electronics and Embedded Systems Engineering (ICCNEEE), IEEE (Institute of Electrical and Electronics Engineers, Inc.). 2015. pp. 388-391

[4] Meng GC, Shahzad A, Saad NM, Malik AS, Meriaudeau F. Prototype design for wearable veins localization system using near infrared imaging technique. In: 2015 IEEE 11th International Colloquium on Signal Processing & Its Applications (CSPA), Haidawati Mohamad Nasir. 2015. pp. 112-115

[5] Wang Y-H, Hung C-J, Shen C-H, Chen S-J. A new oxygen saturation images of iris tissue. In: 2010 IEEE Sensors, IEEE (Institute of Electrical and Electronics Engineers, Inc.). 2010. pp. 1386-1389

[6] Ye Z, Luo J, Bhattacharya P. Optimal approach for enhancement of large and small scale near-infrared and infrared imaging. In: 2005 International Conference on Industrial Electronics and Control Applications, IEEE (Institute of Electrical and Electronics Engineers, Inc.). 2005. p. 6

[7] Berezin MY, Lee H, Akers W, Guo K, Goiffon RJ, Almutairi A, et al. Engineering NIR dyes for fluorescent lifetime contrast. In: 2009 Annual International Conference of the IEEE Engineering in Medicine and Biology Society, IEEE (Institute of Electrical and Electronics Engineers, Inc.). 2009. pp. 114-117

[8] Gan KB, Zahedi E, Ali MAM. Transabdominal fetal heart rate detection using NIRPhotopleythysmography: Instrumentation and clinical results. IEEE Transactions on Biomedical Engineering. IEEE (Institute of Electrical and Electronics Engineers, Inc.). 2009;**56**(8):2075-2082

[9] Alacam B, Yazici B. Direct reconstruction of pharmacokinetic-rate images of optical fluorophores from NIR measurements. IEEE Transactions on Medical Imaging. IEEE (Institute of Electrical and Electronics Engineers, Inc.). 2009;**28**(9):1337-1353

[10] Soraghan CJ, Ward TE, Matthews F, Markham C. Optical safety assessment of a near-infrared brain-computer interface. In: IET Irish Signals and Systems Conference (ISSC 2008). 2008. pp. 174-179

[11] Wieringa FP, Mastik F, Duncker DJGM, Bogers AJJC, Zeelenberg C, van, der Steen AFW. Remote optical stereoscopic multispectral imaging during cardiac surgery. In: 2006 Computers in Cardiology. 2006. pp. 693-696

[12] Nikolic K, Grossman N, Yan H, Drakakis E, Toumazou C, Degenaar

P. A non-invasive retinal prosthesis—Testing the concept. In: 29th Annual International Conference of the IEEE Engineering in Medicine and Biology Society, IEEE (Institute of Electrical and Electronics Engineers, Inc.). 2007. pp. 6364-6367

[13] Sao V, Pourrezaei K, Akin A, Ayaz H. Breast tumor imaging using NIR LED based handheld continuous-wave imager. In: IEEE 29th Annual Proceedings of Bioengineering Conference, IEEE (Institute of Electrical and Electronics Engineers, Inc.). 2003. pp. 55-56

[14] Colak SB, van der Mark MB, Hooft GWT, Hoogenraad JH, van der Linden ES, Kuijpers FA. Clinical optical tomography and NIR spectroscopy for breast cancer detection. IEEE Journal of Selected Topics in Quantum Electronics. 1999;5(4):1143-1158

[15] Yavas S, Kipergil EA, Uluc N, Demirkiran A, Kayikcioglu T, Salman HS, et al. Optical resolution photoacoustic imaging of multiple probes via single fiber laser with independently adjustable parameters. In: 2017 Conference on Lasers and Electro-Optics Europe & European Quantum Electronics Conference (CLEO/Europe-EQEC), IEEE (Institute of Electrical and Electronics Engineers, Inc.). 2017. pp. 1-1

[16] Kim S, Choi Y, Kim KB. Realtime intraoperative imaging system combining annihilation γ-ray detectors and video projectors. In: 2015 IEEE Nuclear Science Symposium and Medical Imaging Conference (NSS/MIC), IEEE (Institute of Electrical and Electronics Engineers, Inc.). 2015. pp. 1-1

[17] Abdeladl O, Schleicher M, Portilla M, Shaporev A, Reukov V. Development of a portable near infrared camera for early detection of diabetic ulcers. In: 2016 32nd Southern Biomedical Engineering Conference (SBEC), IEEE (Institute of Electrical and Electronics Engineers, Inc.). 2016. pp. 55-56

[18] Lawand K, Parihar M, Shital N, Patil. Design and development of infrared LED based non invasive blood glucometer. In: 2015 Annual IEEE India Conference (INDICON), IEEE (Institute of Electrical and Electronics Engineers, Inc.). 2015. pp. 1-6

[19] Noh ZM, Ramli AR, Saripan MI, Hanafi M. Assessment of near infrared LED radiation pattern using Otsu thresholding. In: 2015 IEEE Student Symposium in Biomedical Engineering & Sciences (ISSBES), IEEE (Institute of Electrical and Electronics Engineers, Inc.). 2015. pp. 1-6

[20] Daianu M, Mezher A, Jahanshad N, Hibar DP, Nir TM, Jack CR, et al. Spectral graph theory and graph energy metrics show evidence for the alzheimer's disease disconnection syndrome in APOE-4 risk gene carriers. In: 2015 IEEE 12th International Symposium on Biomedical Imaging (ISBI), IEEE (Institute of Electrical and Electronics Engineers, Inc.). 2015. pp. 458-461

[21] Gioux S. Clinical translation of near-infrared image-guided surgery: Where do we stand? In: 2014 Conference on Lasers and Electro-Optics (CLEO)—Laser Science to Photonic Applications, Optical Society of America. 2014. pp. 1-1

[22] Unnikrishna Menon KA, Hemachandran D, Abhishek TK. A survey on non-invasive blood glucose monitoring using NIR. In: 2013 International Conference on Communication and Signal Processing, IEEE (Institute of Electrical and Electronics Engineers, Inc.). 2013. pp. 1069-1072

[23] Tsai H-Y, Huang K-C, Chang H-C, Chang C-H. A study on oxygen saturation images constructed from the skin tissue of human hand. In: 2013 IEEE International Instrumentation and Measurement Technology Conference, IEEE (Institute of Electrical and Electronics Engineers, Inc.). (I2MTC). 2013. pp. 58-62

[24] Roche R, Jung YJ, Godavarty A. Implementation of a novel, integrative approach for optical 3D positional tracking towards accurate co-registered imaging using hand-held optical imagers. In: 2013 29th Southern Biomedical Engineering Conference, IEEE (Institute of Electrical and Electronics Engineers, Inc.). 2013. pp. 81-82

[25] Huang K-C, Chang C-L, Chang H-C, Chang C-H. The image analysis of skin tissue irradiated with difference wavelengths of LED sources. In: 2012 IEEE International Instrumentation and Measurement Technology Conference Proceedings, IEEE (Institute of Electrical and Electronics Engineers, Inc.). 2012. pp. 1246-1250

[26] Kalkstein N, Kinar Y, Na'aman M, Neumark N, Akiva P. Using machine learning to detect problems in ECG data collection. In: 2011 Computing in Cardiology, IEEE (Institute of Electrical and Electronics Engineers, Inc.). 2011. pp. 437-440

[27] Fabila DA, de la Rosa JM, Stolik S, Moreno E, Dominguez J, Mercado SM, et al. Portable system for measuring fluorescence signals of biological tissue. IEEE Latin America Transactions. IEEE (Institute of Electrical and Electronics Engineers, Inc.). 2011;**9**(7):1012-1017

[28] Sultan E, Khwaja A, Manseta K, Mallalah Y, Zhang Q Najafizadeh L, et al. Comparison of tethered and untethered helmet mounted fNIR systems for TBI application. In: WAMICON 2011 Conference Proceedings, IEEE (Institute of Electrical and Electronics Engineers, Inc.). 2011. pp. 1-4

[29] Benaron DA, Lenox M, Goheen M, Stevenson DK. Noninvasive measurement and imaging of tissue structure and oxygenation using infrared time-of-flight absorbance (TOFA) spectrophotometry. In: 1992 14th Annual International Conference of the IEEE Engineering in Medicine and Biology Society, IEEE (Institute of Electrical and Electronics Engineers, Inc.). Vol. 6. 1992. pp. 2404-2406

[30] Trabelsi A, Boukadoum M, Siaj M. Blood glucose optical bio-implant: Preliminary design guidelines. In: 2010 Biomedical Circuits and Systems Conference (BioCAS), IEEE (Institute of Electrical and Electronics Engineers, Inc.). 2010. pp. 150-153

[31] Degenaar P, McGovern B, Berlinguer-Palmini R, Vysokov N, Grossman N, Pohrer V, et al. Individually addressable optoelectronic arrays for optogenetic neural stimulation. In: 2010 Biomedical Circuits and Systems Conference (BioCAS),IEEE (Institute of Electrical and Electronics Engineers, Inc.). 2010. pp. 170-173

Chapter 5

Telerobotic 3D Articulated Arm-Assisted Surgery Tools with Augmented Reality for Surgery Training

Ahmad Hoirul Basori and Hani Moaiteq Abdullah AlJahdali

Abstract

In this research, human body will be marked and tracked using depth camera. The arm motion from the trainer will be sent through network and then mapped into 3D robotic arm in the destination server. The robotic arm will move according to the trainer. In the meantime, trainee will follow the movement and they can learn how to do particular tasks according to the trainer. The telerobotic-assisted surgery tools will give guidance how to slice or do simple surgery in several steps through the 3D medical images which are displayed in the human body. User will do training and selects some of the body parts and then analyzes it. The system provide specific task to be completed during training and measure how many tasks the user can accomplish during the surgical time. The telerobotic-assisted virtual surgery tools using augmented reality (AR) is expected to be used widely in medical education as an alternative system with low-cost solution.

Keywords: telerobotics, augmented reality, 3D medical images, robotic arm, virtual surgery

1. Introduction

The study of robot controlled to follow certain paths by considering the collision with surrounding object has been studied extensively for the past years. The robot is usually manipulated through a particular device. In order to adjust the robot movement, user should reprogram the microcontroller that is attached to the robot to do certain task.

Robotic arm is one of the robotic parts, which is widely used for several fields including in the medical rehabilitation to assist a disable people. Implementing the real 3D arm is quite costly; the 3D simulated articulated robotic arm is offering new ways of simulation. In addition, the gesture tracking also offers the natural ways of interaction by providing the real-time synchronization between human arm and 3D arm.

Kinect was originally invented as a device for game; however, it also can be used for other purposes such as helping the recovery process of patient who got stroke. The doctor can monitor the improvement of patient and trail their nerve movement. By investigating the nerve of a person's skeletal connection, healing specialists will have competency to find zones of body parts that requires intense training. The response that person acquired throughout or subsequently through a rehabilitation period is still possible to be perfected to solve precise badly behaved zones for the patient's movement. The Kinect has a possibility as rehabilitation tools in house. Rehabilitation in the house provides suppleness for the patient to do regular reiteration of therapy.

Furthermore, to motivate neuron recurrence inside human mind that manipulates body change, therapy should be repetitive for a period of time. Idea behind the interface is that new position commands for the robot will be derived from the depth map captured by the Kinect. The interface offers methods to start and stop the Kinect, translate points from the Kinect's position to robot's position, and retrieve the latest position calculated by the Kinect. The control algorithm which is able to find the next position of the robot and, so that he/she can get exactly the wanted functionality. The Kinect uses a few seconds to start and to calibrate itself to give accurate depth measurements, so it is recommended that the Kinect interface is initialized at the same time as the robot system is turned on.

Most of the devices that used in hospital are really costly, and the procedure can be so complicated. They require very strict permission with authorized personnel to run the device and the queue can be quite long. Furthermore, some researchers focus on studying the communication between patient and therapist by providing the remote access through network to do home-based therapy [1]. In addition, the training system for elderly is also being studied to provide better design for attractive training system, since it can be conducted in home personally [2].

Augmented reality is also widely used for helping people on finding the path/route for pilgrim by combining AR technology and GPS trackers [3–6]. In addition, the telecommunication in medical field such as telemedicine also has strong correlation with brain computer interface and haptic technology that increases the realism of telemedicine technology. The virtual character that assists the user will do their best to imitate human behavior as well as their interaction among themselves that will strive collision response in virtual environment [7–15]. With advanced collision handling, it will also reflect the realism of interaction between user and virtual agent [15]. Besides, researcher also studied the hand and finger tracking to assist doctor on viewing and manipulating the 3D model of human body [16, 17]. While another research try to improve augmented or virtual reality technology by producing realistic facial expression in the conventional teaching system [18].

2. Research method

2.1 Research methodology

The process is initiated by placing the Kinect camera in front of the user and then adjusting the optimum distance for acquiring finest depth image. Subsequently, it will capture the human body, which is then transferred into depth image stream. The second phase is random decision forest algorithm application by choosing a set of threshold for segmentation. The threshold and attribute which have high-density information are chosen and then the process is repeated. The final phase is mapping between joint skeleton and robotic arms and then starting the simulation by controlling remotely.

The methodology of the project consists of three main processes as shown in **Figure 1**.

Figure 1 describes that the telerobotic arm was initiated by placing the depth camera in front of the user to capture the human body and produce a stream of depth image. The algorithm used here is random decision forest that can determine the arm position of human body in real time. The process will be repeated until the desired accuracy has been satisfied. There are two vectors that built joint direction.

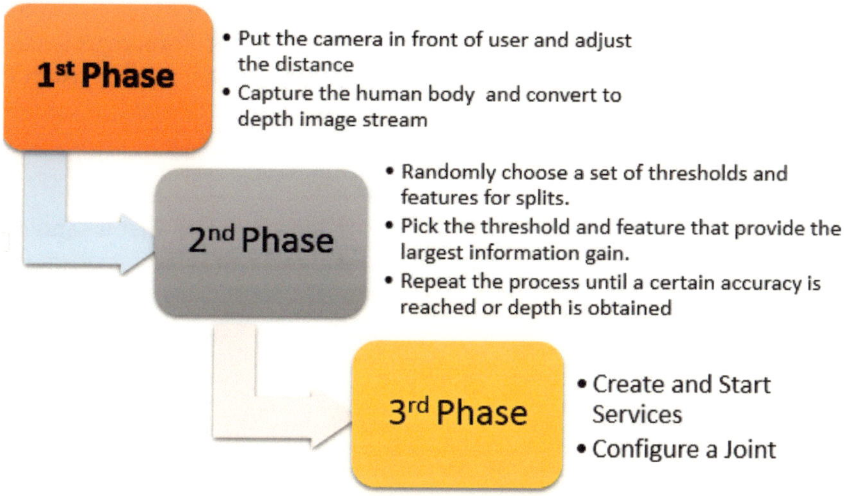

Figure 1.
Project methodology.

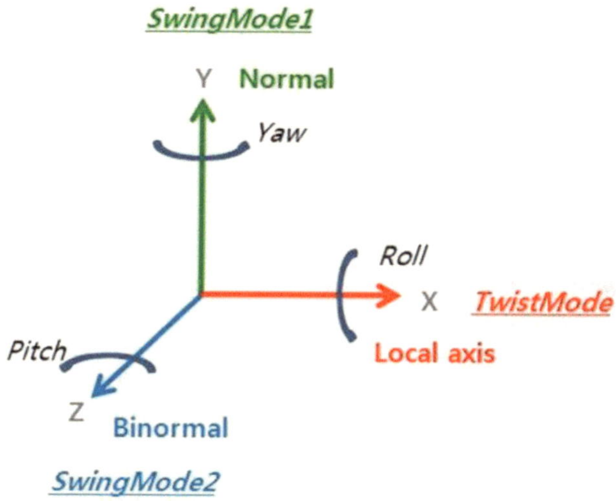

Figure 2.
Join frame diagram.

Three axes, which define the joint frame, are the local or joint axis, the normal axis, and the binormal axis as shown in **Figure 2**.

2.2 Result of software requirement

The proposed application provides some features for user to interact with the system that is classified as functional and nonfunctional requirement as listed below:

2.2.1 Functional requirement

2.2.1.1 Gesture tracking

Gesture recognition can be divided into four main phases: hand movement detection, classifying the gesture from a collection of images, pull out the characteristic and then distinguish the gesture. The hand motion is determined through color of the skin and movement analysis. The speed of hand motion is computed to interpret the gesture localization from repeated images. Therefore, by collecting the depth images and analyzing the images, it can stimulate meaningful gestures that contain a particular command.

2.2.1.2 Real-time feedback

The real-time feedback is provided with depth image stream that is send out by Kinect and then analyzed using random forest algorithm. The algorithm will produce a skeleton joint that will be mapped into 3D robotic arm remotely.

2.2.2 Nonfunctional requirement

2.2.2.1 Finger tracking

The finger tracking is not covered in this research due to its complexity and it requires very short distance during tracking process while gesture requires a longer distance.

2.2.2.2 Full body synchronization

The robotic arm does not need full body tracking and synchronization because the system will focus on the arm of human.

2.3 Use case diagram

Figure 3 shows the use case diagram of the system. There are three main use cases: Kinect sensor, 3D articulated arm, and 3D arm control.

2.3.1 Actor description

The actor of the above system represents the patient or other users who interact with the arm robot system

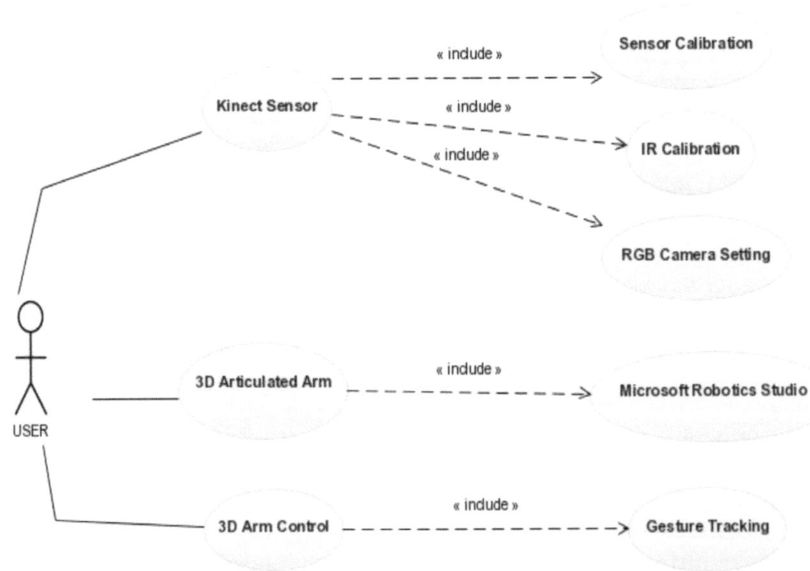

Figure 3.
Use case diagram.

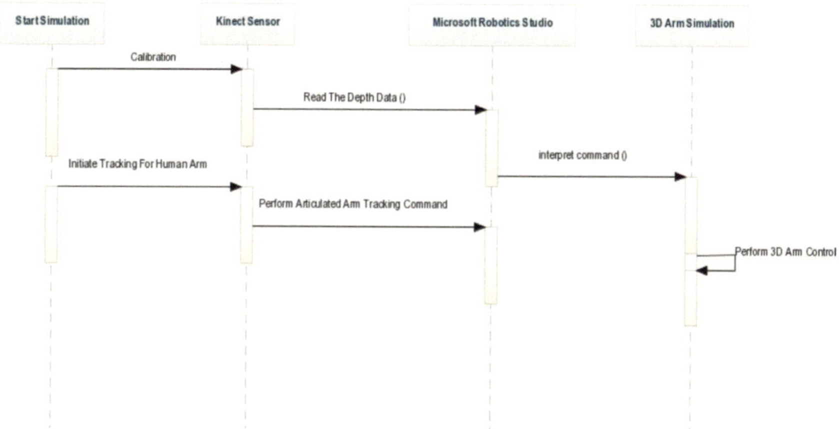

Figure 4.
Sequence diagram.

2.3.2 Use case description

The Kinect sensor is a motion-sensing controller that is able to sense user arm in motion mode. The Kinect needs sensor calibration before it is used, and the Kinect is able to detect depth by using an IR camera. The 3D articulated arm communicates with Microsoft Robotic Studio, while 3D arm control with gesture tracking.

2.4 Analysis phase

This section describes the sequence of project phases such as sequence diagram, activity diagram, and architecture of the system.

2.4.1 Sequence diagram

Figure 4 shows the sequence process of the system that starts with simulation and calibration with Kinect sensor and then it is continued by reading the depth data of user arm. Microsoft Robotic Studio will render the 3D arm and is synchronized with interpreted command of 3D arm and then performs 3D arm control.

2.4.2 Activity diagram

Figures 5 and **6** show two activity diagrams: diagram (A) is started with simulation, adjusting distance, tracking, capturing human depth image, and then classifying gesture.

While the activity diagram in **Figure 6** starts with gesture classification, joint classification, than joint synchronization between human joint with 3D arm joint, and provide real time interaction between 3D articulated arm.

2.5 Architecture design phase

Figure 7 depicts the architecture design phase that has Kinect sensor component, and the other component is Microsoft Robotic Simulator that has capability to connect with Kinect driver and Kinect software development kit (SDK). Microsoft Robotic Studio consists of visual programming language and 3D environment model.

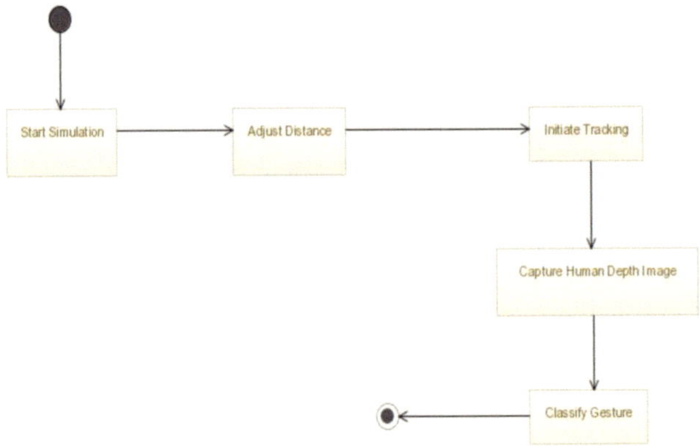

Figure 5.
Activity diagram (A).

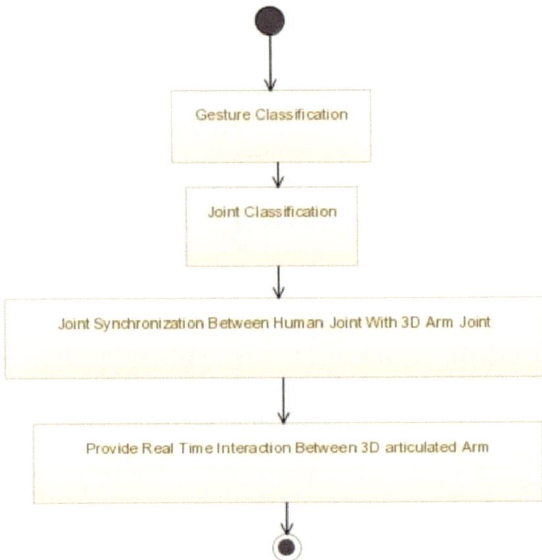

Figure 6.
Activity diagram (B).

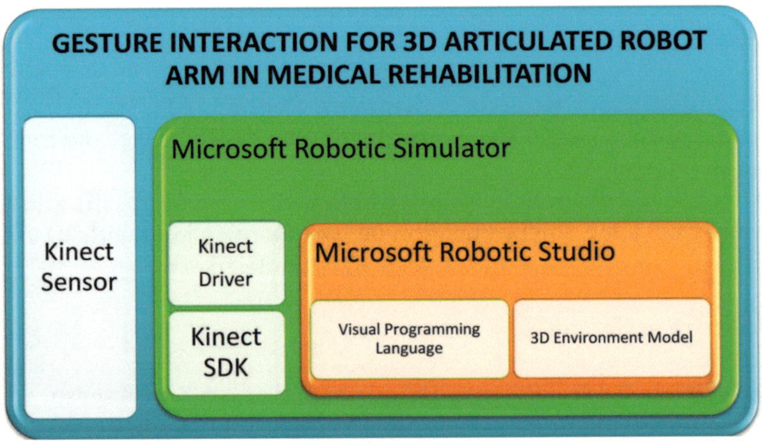

Figure 7.
Architecture design phase diagram.

3. Result and discussion

The first testing shows how to manage the tracker for hand control; it is started by initiating the Kinect camera to capture the human joint and render 3D hand that will follow the mouse movement.

3.1 Hand tracking control

The hand tracking control is used for motion detection of human hand as shown in **Figure 8.** The system is to track and differentiate right hand or left hand of human. **Figure 9** is the result of robotic arm rotation using Kinect gesture.

Figures 10 and **11** also demonstrate the movement of joint of robotic arm using Kinect gesture. The robotic arm will move according to the joint data that are sent through network by following the trainer movement remotely.

3.2 Performance testing

The performance of rendering is satisfying when the frame per second (FPS) is very high and the highest score reaches 60 while the lowest is 54, as shown in **Figure 12**.

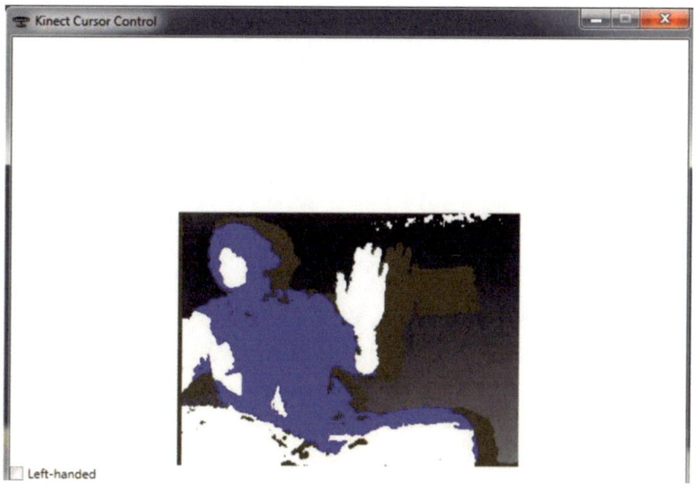

Figure 8.
Kinect depth camera tracking human hand.

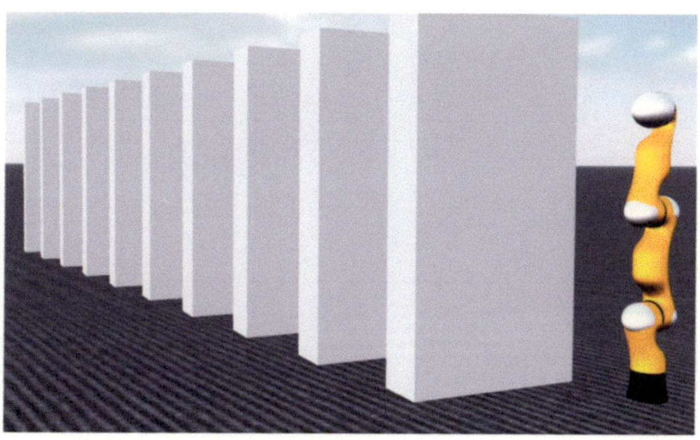

Figure 9.
Robotics arm which is connected to Kinect in steady position with domino blocks.

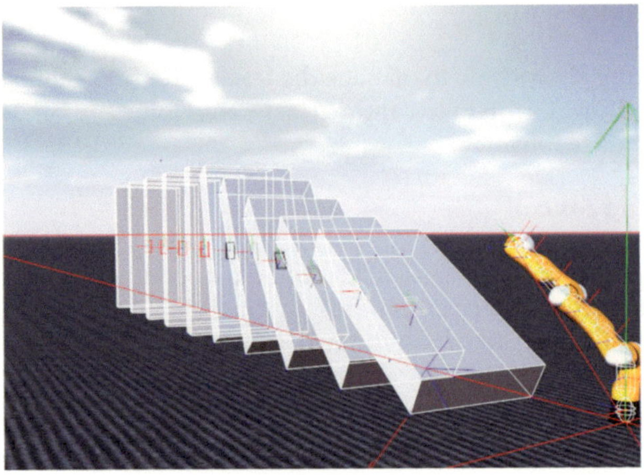

Figure 10.
User controlling the robotic arm to hit the blocks of domino.

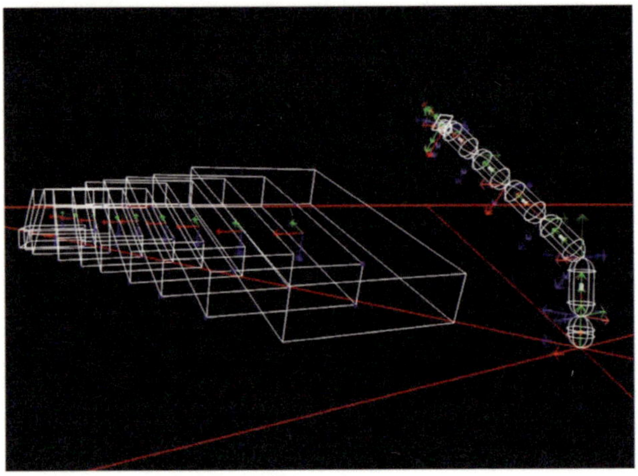

Figure 11.
Robotics arm in wireframe mode.

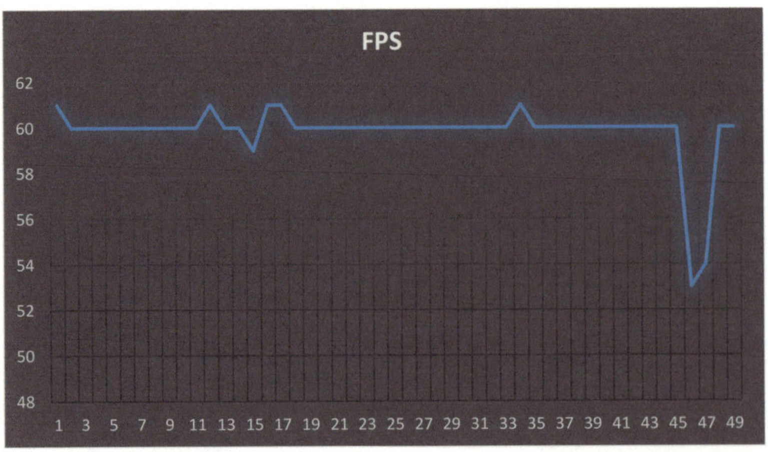

Figure 12.
The statistical measurement of frame rate per second.

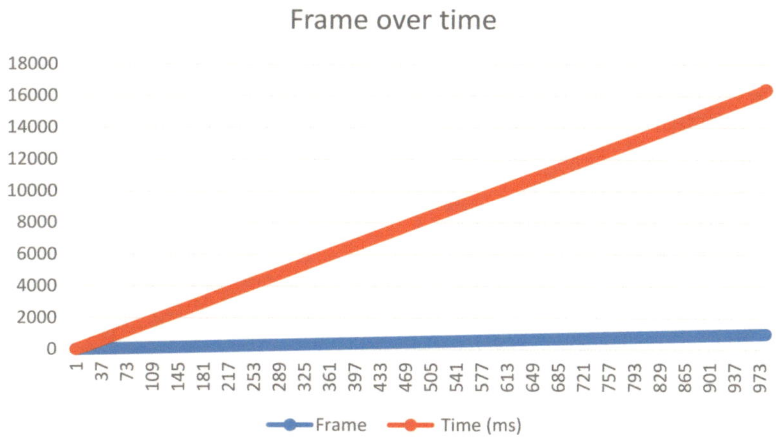

Figure 13.
The statistical measurement of frame over time.

Frames	Time (ms)	Min	Max	Avg
982	16,411	55	61	59.838
1935	33,119	5	61	58.426
99	1638	59	61	60.44

Table 1.
Frame, time, max, and average.

Figure 13 and **Table 1** also portray the statistical measurement of the rendering process of 3D articulated robotic arm during the testing.

4. Conclusions

Telerobotic is one of the essential research topics, which is widely applied into medical rehabilitation and even manufacturing process in industry. This paper aims to provide telerobotic arm with six joints that represent human arm. This arm can be rotated and can act like human arm. The idea of the project is to provide training or exercise for poststroke patient to move their hand by controlling the 3D articulated arm. The human hand is tracked down by depth camera, and the behavior of real hand and 3D Arm is synchronized in real time. In this project, we provide five joints of 3D robotic arms that can be rotated according to its angle. The 3D arms will be simulated with domino effect when they collide with each other. The user will control the arm by performing a gesture in front of Kinect camera, and the synchronization of joints between human arm and 3D arm is performed in real time. The control process through Kinect by imitating mouse cursor movement also runs smoothly during the testing process. This finding is believed to bring potential benefits to rehabilitation for certain patients such as poststroke rehabilitation. The result is very convincing, while interaction is conducted naturally just by waving their hands or rotating the joints of our hand, 3D arm will do rotation as well. For future recommendation, the result of project can be improved further by conducting clinical test to real patient in medical rehabilitation and it can be used as a simulator in manufacturing process in industries.

Acknowledgements

This work was supported by the deanship of scientific research (DSR), King Abdulaziz University, and Jeddah Saudi Arabia. The authors, therefore, gratefully acknowledge the DSR for technical and financial support.

Author details

Ahmad Hoirul Basori* and Hani Moaiteq Abdullah AlJahdali
Faculty of Computing and Information Technology Rabigh, King Abdulaziz University, Saudi Arabia

*Address all correspondence to: abasori@kau.edu.sa

References

[1] Anton D, Kurillo G, Goñi A, Illarramendi A, Bajcsy R. Real-time communication for Kinect-based telerehabilitation. Future Generation Computer Systems. 2017;**75**:72-81

[2] Ofli F, Kurillo G, Obdržálek Š, Bajcsy R, Jimison HB, Pavel M. Design and evaluation of an interactive exercise coaching system for older adults: Lessons learned. IEEE Journal of Biomedical and Health Informatics. 2016;**20**(1):201-212

[3] Afif FN, Basori AH, Saari N. Vision based tracking technology for augmented reality: A survey. International Journal of Interactive Digital Media. 2013;**1**(1):46-49

[4] Afif FN, Basori AH, Almazyad AS, et al. Fast markerless tracking for augmented reality in planar environment. Procedia - Social and Behavioral Sciences. 2013;**97**(6): 648-655

[5] Basori AH, Afif FN. Orientation control for indoor virtual landmarks based on hybrid-based markerless augmented reality. 3D Research. 2015;**6**:41. DOI: 10.1007/s13319-015-0072-5

[6] Albaqami NN, Allehaibi KH, Basori AH. Augmenting pilgrim experience and safety with geo-location way finding and mobile augmented reality. International Journal of Computer Science and Network Security. 2018;**18**(2):23-32

[7] Basori AH et al. The feasibility of human haptic emotion as a feature to enhance interactivity and immersiveness on virtual reality game. In: Proceedings of the 7th ACM SIGGRAPH International Conference on Virtual-Reality Continuum and Its Applications in Industry. Singapore: ACM; 2008. pp. 1-2

[8] Basori AH, Qasim AZ. Extreme expression of sweating in 3D virtual human. Computers in Human Behavior. 2014;**35**:307-314. DOI: 10.1016/j.chb.2014.03.013

[9] Basori AH, Ahmed MA, PrabuwonoAS YA, Bramantoro A, Syamsuddin I, Alehaibi KH. Profound correlation of human and NAO-robot interaction through facial expression controlled by EEG sensor. International Journal of Advanced and Applied Science. 2018;**5**:8. DOI: 10.21833/ijaas.2018.08.013

[10] Basori AH. Emotion walking for humanoid avatars using brain signals. International Journal of Advanced Robotic Systems; **10**:1-11. DOI: 10.5772/54764. http://journals.sagepub.com/doi/abs/10.5772/54764

[11] Ahmed MAK, Basori AH. The influence of beta signal toward emotion classification for facial expression control through EEG sensors. Procedia - Social and Behavioral Sciences. Elsevier; 2013. DOI: 10.1016/j.sbspro.2013.10.294

[12] Basori AH, Bade A, Sunar MS, Daman D, Saari N, Salam MDH. An integration framework of haptic feedback to improve facial expression. International Journal of Innovative Computing, Information and Control (IJICIC). 2012;**8**(11):7829-7851

[13] Basori AH, Afif FN, Almazyad AS, Abujabal HA, Rehman A, Alkawaz MH. Fast markerless tracking for augmented reality in planar environment. 3D Research. 2015, 2015;**6**(4):1-11. DOI: 10.1007/s13319-015-0072-5. Article 72

[14] Basori AH, Daman D, Bade A, et al. The feasibility of human haptic emotion as a feature to enhance interactivity and immersiveness on virtual reality game. In: Proceedings of the 7th ACM

SIGGRAPH International Conference on Virtual-Reality Continuum and Its Applications in Industry (VRCAI '08). New York, NY, USA: ACM. Article 37; 2008. 2 pages. DOI: 10.1145/1477862.1477910

[15] Abdullasim N, Basori AH, Salam MD, Bade A. Velocity perception: Collision handling technique for agent avoidance behavior. Telkomnika. 2013;**11**(4):2264-2270

[16] Yusoff MA, Basori AH, Mohamed F. Interactive hand and arm gesture control for 2D medical image and 3D volumetric medical visualization. Procedia - Social and Behavioral Sciences. 2013;**97**:723-729. Elsevier

[17] Suroso MR, Basori AH, Mohamed F. Finger-based gestural interaction for exploration of 3D heart visualization. Procedia - Social and Behavioral Sciences. 2013;**97**:684-690. Elsevier

[18] Basori AH, Tenriawaru A, Mansur ABF. Intelligent avatar on E-learning using facial expression and haptic, TELKOMNIKA (Telecommunication Computing Electronics and Control). 2011;**9**(1):115-124